FIRST
AID
MANUAL

**IRISH
RED CROSS**

**ORDER OF
MALTA AMBULANCE CORPS**

FIRST
AID
MANUAL

The Authorised Manual of
the Irish Red Cross
and the Order of Malta Ambulance Corps

Andrew K Marsden FRCSEd
*Consultant in Accident and Emergency Medicine,
Pinderfields Hospital, Wakefield*

Sir Cameron Moffat KBE HonDSc FRCS
late Royal Army Medical Corps (retd)

Roy Scott DL JP MD FRCSGlas FRCSEd
Consultant Urologist, Royal Infirmary, Glasgow

DORLING KINDERSLEY
LONDON • NEW YORK • STUTTGART

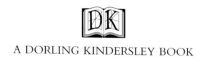

A DORLING KINDERSLEY BOOK

Sixth edition first published in Great Britain in 1992 by
Dorling Kindersley Limited, 9 Henrietta Street, Covent Garden,
London WC2E 8PS.
Reprinted in 1993 and 1995

A CIP catalogue record for this book is available from
the British Library

ISBN 0-90607-704-4

FOREWORD

The pace and complexity of modern living has resulted in a growing number of accidental injuries – this despite increased safety controls.

The Barrington Commission on Health and Saftety at Work estimated that up to 250,000 injuries requiring first aid occur each year in the Irish workplace. The accident figures for the wider community – homes, sportsfields, and transport – are likely to be even more alarming.

The need for improved emergency first aid care comes from both the public and the state. The Hamilton Report on safety in public places, the Health and Safety Authority regulations on First Aid in the Workplace, and the current upgrading of the nation's ambulance service all point to the need for better first aid arrangements.

This new sixth edition of the *First Aid Manual* will help address that need. Now fully revised and updated in line with recent medical developments, this manual is the authoritative guide to first aid. It serves as both a reference and an instructional text. Its simple, problem-centred approach will guarantee a wide appeal.

First aid is largely a skill requiring supervised practice and training and is best learned at an approved course.

For details of First Aid Courses in your area, please contact your local Red Cross Branch.

Irish Red Cross 1995

CONTENTS

INTRODUCTION

This new edition of the First Aid Manual has been completely revised and re-written, making the information it contains completely up to date and consistent with current medical thought. The recommendations for resuscitation techniques in particular now follow standards set by the European Resuscitation Council and the American Heart Association.

Other changes have been made in order to make the First Aid Manual more accessible and useful, not just for regular First Aiders, but for all caring citizens. The subject matter has been re-organised, and an ingenious use of colour-coding, coupled with clear cross-referencing, makes information quick and easy to find. A new quick-reference section covering common emergencies is placed at the back of the book for instant access.

More emphasis is laid throughout on human concerns, including those of the First Aider: what you can and should do, and what you should not do; what the casualty may be experiencing; and what your own feelings and reactions may be when called upon to act in stressful situations. Less space is given to those aspects of first aid, such as transportation, that are covered in depth by training courses. Useful new chapters draw together common everyday ailments and injuries that may occur at home, at work, at leisure, and during foreign travel.

Every skill is enhanced by a wider understanding of its subject. In each chapter of this new edition, panelled information tells you more about how the body works, and what may go wrong to produce the group of illnesses or injuries under discussion.

The First Aid Manual also addresses specific problems of our times – for example, Aids, drink- and drug-related disorders, even legal concerns – in a manner which, it is hoped, will dispel modern-day anxieties and prejudice in a safe and sensible way.

How to use the book

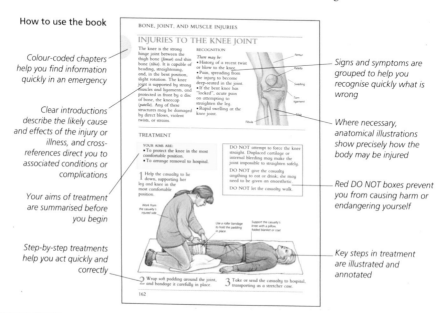

Colour-coded chapters help you find information quickly in an emergency

Clear introductions describe the likely cause and effects of the injury or illness, and cross-references direct you to associated conditions or complications

Your aims of treatment are summarised before you begin

Step-by-step treatments help you act quickly and correctly

Signs and symptoms are grouped to help you recognise quickly what is wrong

Where necessary, anatomical illustrations show precisely how the body may be injured

Red DO NOT boxes prevent you from causing harm or endangering yourself

Key steps in treatment are illustrated and annotated

WHAT IS FIRST AID?

First aid is the initial assistance or treatment given to a casualty for any injury or sudden illness before the arrival of an ambulance, doctor, or other qualified person.

Being a First Aider

Most people can, by following the guidance given in this book, give useful and effective first aid. However, the term "First Aider" is usually applied to someone who has completed a course of theoretical and practical instruction, and passed a professionally supervised examination.

First aid qualifications

The standard First Aid Certificate, awarded by the Irish Red Cross Society, is proof of all-round competence. It is valid for only three years; to keep your knowledge and skills up to date, you must be re-examined after further training. Regular First Aiders may volunteer for additional training to broaden the scope of their skills.

THE AIMS OF FIRST AID:

- To preserve life.
- To limit the effects of the condition.
- To promote recovery.

THE FIRST AIDER IS:

- Highly trained.
- Examined and regularly re-examined.
- Up to date in knowledge and skill.

BEING A FIRST AIDER

The first aid you learn from a manual or course is not quite like reality. Most of us feel some apprehension when faced with "the real thing" – even doctors have qualms when faced with difficult cases. By facing up to these feelings, we are better able to cope with the unexpected.

Doing your best

First aid is a skill based on knowledge, training, and experience. It is not an exact science, and is thus open to human error and circumstances beyond our control. You must accept that however appropriate your treatment, and however hard you try, a casualty may not respond as expected, and may even die. Some conditions inevitably lead to death, even in the best medical hands. Providing you do your best, and what you believe to be correct, your conscience can be clear.

Weighing up the risks

While following the golden rule, "First do no harm", you must also accept the principle of the "calculated risk". Even if there is some risk, it is right to apply a treatment that should benefit the majority of casualties. You must not, however, use a doubtful treatment just for the sake of doing *something*.

Being criticised

First Aiders often express fears of doing something wrong, and even being sued. The "Good Samaritan" principle supports those acting in an emergency (though it will not protect those who stray beyond accepted boundaries). If you keep your head, and follow the guidelines laid out in this book, you need not fear any legal consequences.

Responsibilities of a First Aider

• To assess a situation quickly and safely, and summon appropriate help.
• To identify, as far as possible, the injury or the nature of the illness affecting a casualty.
• To give early, appropriate, and adequate treatment in a sensible order of priority.
• To arrange for the removal of the casualty to hospital, to the care of a doctor, or home.
• To remain with a casualty until handing him or her over to the care of an appropriate person.
• To make and pass on a report, and give further help if required.

More information concerning first aid requirements at work and in public places can be found on page 232.

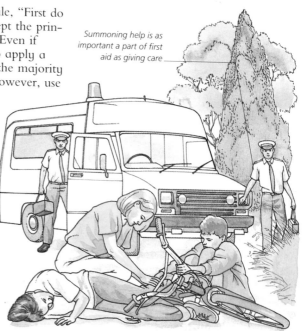

Summoning help is as important a part of first aid as giving care

GIVING CARE WITH CONFIDENCE

Every casualty needs to feel secure and in safe hands. You can create a beneficial atmosphere of confidence and assurance by:

- Being in control, both of yourself and the problem.
- Acting calmly and logically.
- Being gentle, but firm, with your hands, and speaking to the casualty kindly, but purposefully.

Building up trust

Talk to the casualty throughout your examination and treatment:

- Explain what you are going to do.
- Try to answer questions honestly to allay fears as best you can. If you do not know the answer, say so.
- Continue to reassure the casualty even when your treatment is complete – find out about next-of-kin, or anyone else who should be contacted about the incident. Ask if you can help to make arrangements so that any responsibilities the casualty may have – for example, collecting a child from school – can be taken care of.
- Do not leave someone whom you believe to be dying. Continue to talk to the casualty, and hold his or her hands – never let the casualty feel alone.

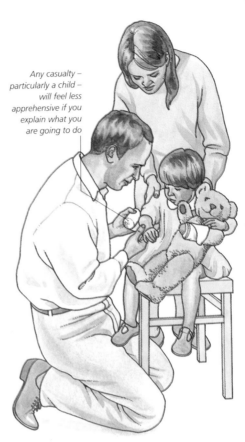

Any casualty – particularly a child – will feel less apprehensive if you explain what you are going to do

Telling relatives

Though informing relatives of a death is the job of the police or a doctor, it may well be that you have to tell family members that someone has been taken ill, or involved in an accident.

Always check first that you are speaking to the right person. Then explain, as simply and honestly as you can, what has happened, and, if appropriate, where the casualty has been taken.

Do not beat about the bush, or exaggerate; you may cause undue alarm. It is better to admit ignorance than to give misleading information.

Coping with children

Young children are extremely perceptive and will quickly detect any uncertainty on your part. Gain an injured or sick child's confidence by talking first to someone he or she trusts – a parent if possible. If the parent accepts you and believes you will help, this confidence will be conveyed to the child.

It is important that a child understands what is happening and what you intend to do – explain as simply as you can, and do not talk over his or her head. Do not separate a child from its mother, father, or other trusted person.

LOOKING AFTER YOURSELF

Giving first aid can be dangerous. Always be watchful for your personal safety. Do not put yourself at risk by attempting heroic rescues in hazardous circumstances.

First Aiders may also be anxious about the possibility of picking up serious infectious diseases from casualties. It is reassuring to note that there are no cases on record of the virus infections hepatitis B or HIV being passed on through giving mouth-to-mouth resuscitation, despite there being a small theoretical risk. However, you must be aware that such conditions may be spread by blood-to-blood contact.

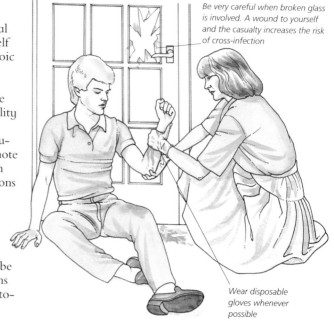

Be very careful when broken glass is involved. A wound to yourself and the casualty increases the risk of cross-infection

Wear disposable gloves whenever possible

Seeking immunisation

If you become concerned that you might have caught something after you have given first aid, contact your doctor. Regular First Aiders should seek medical advice about immunisation against hepatitis B. Protection by immunisation can also sometimes be offered following exposure.

Coping with unpleasantness

The practice of first aid is sometimes messy, smelly, and distasteful, and you may be afraid that you will not be able to cope with unpleasantness. In the event, such fears are usually groundless, and most people perform very well. Taking a first aid course will, however, greatly improve your confidence and self-reliance. The thorough training you will receive will help you to control your emotions, and carry you through many difficult situations.

Taking stock after an emergency

Having given first aid and handed your casualty over, take stock of your own feelings. These may well have been put to one side as you took action, but assisting at an emergency is a stressful event, and it is not uncommon for a "delayed reaction" to strike the First Aider some time afterwards.

Hopefully, your feelings will be of satisfaction, or even elation, but it is not uncommon to feel upset, particularly if you have assisted a stranger and you may thus never know the outcome of your efforts.

Above all, never reproach yourself, or bottle up your feelings. It will often help greatly to talk over your experience with a friend, your doctor, or your first aid trainer.

See also: Preventing cross-infection, page 200.

ACTION AT AN EMERGENCY

The process of first aid often begins before any direct person-to-person contact with the casualty. The way that you approach an incident, and the immediate steps you take to make the area safe and get help, can contribute as much to the casualty's survival and ultimate well-being as any subsequent interventions or medical treatment.

What you will find in this chapter

This chapter outlines the basic guidelines to be observed when approaching any potentially hazardous situation. It also tells you what will happen when you call the emergency services, and how you can be of most use when they arrive. The pages that follow give action plans for many common emergency situations, such as road accidents, fires, and drowning.

THE FIRST AIDER SHOULD:

Assess the situation
- Take in what has happened quickly and calmly.
- Look for dangers to yourself and to the casualty.
- Never put yourself at risk.

Make the area safe
- Protect the casualty from danger.
- Do not try to do too much yourself.

Assess all casualties and give emergency aid
- With more than one casualty, follow the findings of your assessments (*see pages 27-29*) to decide treatment priorities.

Get help
- Quickly ensure that any necessary specialist help has been summoned and is on its way.

CONTENTS

FIRST AID AT AN EMERGENCY

At an emergency, any number of things may demand your attention at the same time. If you try to do everything at once, you may easily get side-tracked into non-vital activities. Always work to a plan, bearing in mind the main steps of emergency action – *Assess, Make Safe, Give Emergency Aid,* and *Get Help.*

• Control your feelings.
• Take a moment to think.
• Do not place yourself in danger.
• Use your common sense.
• Do not attempt too much alone.

ASSESS THE SITUATION

Your approach should be brisk, but calm and controlled, so that you can quickly take in as much information as possible. Your priorities are to identify any dangers to yourself, to the casualty, and to bystanders, then to assess the resources available to you and the kind of help you may need. State that you have first aid skills when offering your help. If there are no doctors, nurses, or more experienced people present, calmly take charge. First ask yourself these questions:

• Is there any continuing danger?
• Is anyone's life in immediate danger?
• Are there bystanders who can help?
• Do I need specialist help?

MAKE THE AREA SAFE

The conditions that caused the accident may still be presenting further danger. Remember that you must put your own safety first. You cannot help others if you become a casualty yourself.

Often, very simple measures, such as turning off an electric switch, are enough to make the area safe. Sometimes more complicated procedures are required. Never put yourself and the casualty at further risk by attempting to do too much; be aware of your limitations.

Dealing with ongoing danger

If you cannot eliminate a life-threatening hazard, you must try to put some distance between it and the casualty. First attempt to remove the danger from the casualty. As a last resort, remove the casualty from the danger. In many situations, you will need to obtain specialist help and equipment.

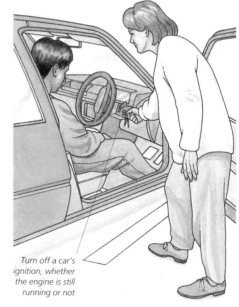

Turn off a car's ignition, whether the engine is still running or not

GIVE EMERGENCY AID

Once it is safe to do so, assess each casualty using the ABC of resuscitation. Your findings will dictate your actions and, if you are on your own, when to get help and the level of help needed. Quickly establish whether the casualty:

- Is fully conscious.
- Is unconscious, but breathing.
- Is not breathing, but has a pulse.
- Has no pulse.

See also: Assessing the casualty, *page 27.*

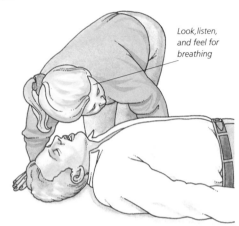

Look, listen, and feel for breathing

> DO NOT delay in summoning any necessary help.

GET HELP

You may be faced with a number of tasks: to maintain safety, to telephone for help (*see overleaf*), and to start giving first aid. Make good use of all your available resources. Other people can be asked to:

- Make the area safe.
- Telephone for assistance.
- Fetch first aid equipment.
- Control traffic and onlookers.
- Control bleeding, or support a limb.
- Maintain the casualty's privacy.
- Help move a casualty to safety.

Give clear instructions and check that they are carried out.

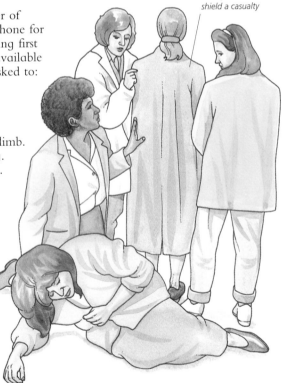

Ask bystanders to shield a casualty

The reactions of onlookers

Do not be upset by bystanders who will not help; there may be good reason why they feel unable to get involved – usually because they have been emotionally affected by the incident. However, giving a bystander a simple task may avert panic or morbid interest, thus helping that person, the casualty, and yourself.

TELEPHONING FOR HELP

You can summon immediate help by telephone from a number of sources, as listed below:
• *Emergency services (999)* Fire, gardai, and ambulance services.
• *Public utilities* Gas, electricity, and water.

• *Health services* Doctor, dentist, nurse, or midwife.
If you are forced to leave a casualty alone, minimise the risks to the casualty by taking any vital action first (*see page 27*). Make your call short but accurate.

FINDING A TELEPHONE

Emergency calls are free, and can be made on any telephone, including car and portable phones. On motorways, emergency telephones can be found every mile; marker posts between them indicate the nearest box. These telephones simply need to be picked up to be answered.

Most large companies have special internal arrangements for calling for assistance. Make sure you are familiar with them.

If you ask someone else to go and make the call, ask him or her to come back and confirm that the call has been made, and that help is on the way.

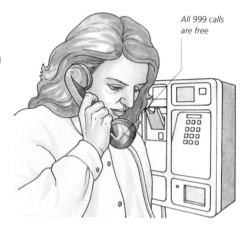

All 999 calls are free

MAKING THE CALL

On dialling 999, you will be asked which service you need, and put through to the appropriate control officer. Whenever there are casualties, ask for the ambulance service; each control can, if necessary, pass on messages to other services.

What the control officer needs to know

Give clear details of the accident or emergency, the number of casualties, and any additional hazards. If you are not sure of your precise location, do not panic – your call can be traced to any call box or motorway telephone.

DO NOT put the telephone down until the control officer clears the line.

Calling the emergency services
Always give the following information:
• Your telephone number.
• The exact location of the incident; a road name or number, if possible, and any junctions or other landmarks.
• The type and seriousness of the incident – for example: "Traffic accident, two cars, road blocked, three people trapped".
• The number, sex, and approximate ages of the casualties, and anything you know about their condition – for example, "Man, early fifties, suspected heart attack, cardiac arrest".
• Details of any hazards such as gas, hazardous substances (*see page 19*), power line damage, or fog.

MULTIPLE CASUALTIES

You may find yourself in the difficult position of having to deal with several casualties at the same time. The order in which you treat them might be crucial to their survival. First attend to anyone who is unconscious. Follow the ABC of resuscitation to establish treatment priority (*see page 27*).

Remember that you can only do your best: you are not expected to make life or death judgements, and will not be criticised if things go badly.

MAJOR INCIDENTS

The characteristics of a major incident are a large number of casualties, the obvious disorder, and therefore the overwhelming demands placed on rescuers.

First, the emergency services need accurate information as to what has happened, so that they can send not only as much help as is needed, but also any specialist personnel or equipment that will aid rescue and treatment. Having ensured that the call has been made, assess the scene and, without putting your safety at risk, start to give emergency aid.

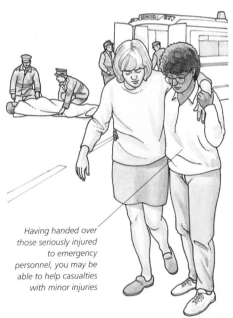

Having handed over those seriously injured to emergency personnel, you may be able to help casualties with minor injuries

When help arrives, the senior emergency services officer will take absolute charge. Usually, the police will control the disaster site, while ambulance officers delegate individuals to various tasks.

The role of the First Aider

Remember that emergency personnel have more on their minds than giving a First Aider "something to do"; do not feel shunned if your offer of help is ignored. More importantly, you *must* leave the incident scene if asked to do so by a member of the emergency services.

However, there are many ways in which you can give valuable assistance – for example, treating minor injuries, or caring for a child whose parent is being treated. Common sense should tell you how you can best be of use.

How you can help

• Casualties with minor injuries should be moved quickly from the site to give clear access to the more serious cases.
• Casualties who are obviously dead should be passed over, so that help can be given to those who need it.
• All those involved should be logged, and casualties tagged, so that accurate records can be made and maintained.
• Workers or residents at or near the site of a disaster should be alerted to security risks and further hazards.
• Any forensic evidence should be carefully preserved.

ROAD ACCIDENTS

Road accidents range from a fall from a bicycle to a major incident with many casualties. Often, the accident site will present serious risks to safety, largely because of oncoming traffic. It is essential to make the area safe – to protect yourself, the casualty, and other road-users.

MAKE THE ACCIDENT SITE SAFE

First ensure your own safety, and that you yourself do not create danger:
• Park safely, well clear of the accident site. Set your hazard lights flashing.
• Do not run across a busy motorway to reach the other side.
• At night, wear or carry something light, or reflective, and use a torch.
Then take these general precautions:
• Send bystanders to warn other drivers.
• Set up warning triangles or lights 200 metres/250 yards in each direction.
• Switch off the ignition of any damaged vehicle and, if you know how, disconnect the battery. Switch off the fuel supply on diesel vehicles and motorcycles.
• Stabilise vehicles. If a vehicle is upright, apply the hand-brake and put it in gear, or put blocks at the wheels. If a vehicle is on its side, do not right it, but try to prevent it from rolling over.
• Look out for physical dangers. Is anyone smoking? Are there goods vehicles displaying Hazchem symbols? Are there damaged power lines, or spilt fuel?

CHECK THE CASUALTIES

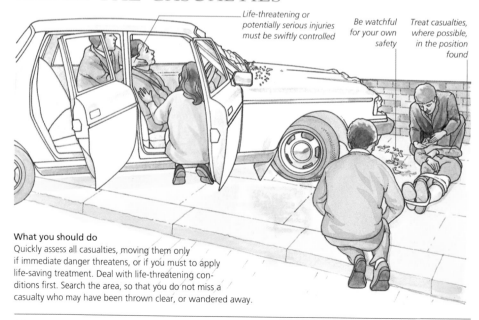

Life-threatening or potentially serious injuries must be swiftly controlled

Be watchful for your own safety

Treat casualties, where possible, in the position found

What you should do
Quickly assess all casualties, moving them only if immediate danger threatens, or if you must to apply life-saving treatment. Deal with life-threatening conditions first. Search the area, so that you do not miss a casualty who may have been thrown clear, or wandered away.

FOR AN UNCONSCIOUS CASUALTY

> DO NOT move the casualty unless it is absolutely necessary.

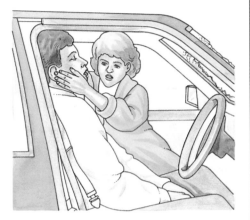

1 Assume there is a neck injury until proved otherwise. Support the casualty's head and neck with your hands, so that he can breathe freely. For additional support, apply a collar, if possible (*see page 155*).

2 Attend to any life-threatening injuries if possible. Observe the casualty continuously until expert help arrives.

IF it is essential to move the casualty, you will need three people to help you: one to support the shoulders and chest, one for the hips and abdomen, and one for the legs. You should support the head continuously, and direct all movements.

FOR A CASUALTY TRAPPED UNDER A VEHICLE

Try to find help to lift or move the vehicle and, if absolutely necessary, drag the casualty clear. Mark the exact position of the vehicle and/or casualty first. The police will need this information.

See also: Crush injuries, *page 92.*

Hazardous substances

Accidents may be complicated by the spillage of dangerous substances or the escape of toxic vapours. Never make any rescue attempt unless you are sure that you are not endangering yourself by coming into contact with a dangerous substance. Keep bystanders well away from the scene, bearing in mind that poisonous fumes may be released and travel some distance. Stand upwind of the accident, so that any fumes are blown away from you.

Coded information for the emergency services   *United Nations number for the substance*

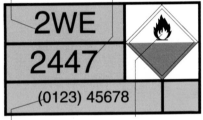

Telephone number for further information   *Nature of potential danger*

Oxidising agents   Poisonous substances   Flammable substances

Radioactive substances   Compressed gases   Corrosive substances

Hazchem symbols
A "Hazchem" placard on a vehicle warns you that it may be carrying a hazardous substance. If you are in any doubt about your safety, or about the meaning of the sign, keep your distance, especially if there is any spillage, or if you see the letter "E" (*as above*). Make a note of the information on the placard and pass it on when telephoning for help.

FIRES

Rapid, clear thinking at a fire is vital. Fire spreads very quickly, so warn any people at risk, and alert the emergency services immediately. Panic also spreads quickly; you must control anyone likely to increase alarm.

Leaving a burning building

Without putting yourself at risk, do your best to help everyone out of a building on fire, shutting doors behind you. Look for notices giving the location of fire exits and assembly points. Familiarise yourself with the guidelines at your workplace or, if you are on business premises as a visitor, follow any instructions given by staff.

See also: Burns and scalds, page 103.

Inhalation of fumes, page 60.

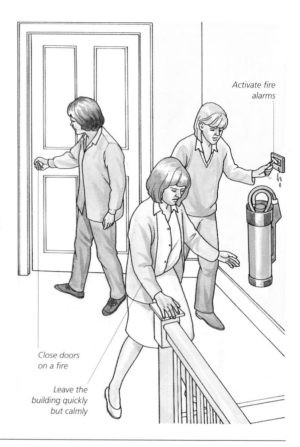

Activate fire alarms

Close doors on a fire

Leave the building quickly but calmly

DEALING WITH A FIRE

A fire needs three components to start it and keep it going: ignition (an electric spark or naked flame); a source of fuel (for example, petrol, wood, or fabrics); and oxygen (air). Remove any one of these, and you break this "triangle of fire". For example:

• *Ignition* Switch off a car's ignition.
• *Fuel* Isolate a vehicle's fuel supply; remove combustible materials, such as curtains, in the path of a fire.
• *Oxygen* Shut doors on a fire; smother flames with an impervious substance.

The triangle of fire
Eliminating any of the three components necessary for combustion will break the triangle and prevent fire.

DO NOT attempt to fight a fire unless you have called the emergency services and made sure that you are not putting your own safety at risk.

SMOKE AND FUME-FILLED AIR

Any fire in a confined space creates a highly dangerous atmosphere that is low in oxygen, and may be contaminated by carbon monoxide and toxic fumes. Never enter a burning or fume-filled building, or open a door leading to a fire. Leave it to the emergency services.

What you can do

● If trapped in a burning building, go into a room with a window and shut the door. If you must pass through a smoke-filled room, keep low down, as the air at floor level is the clearest.

● If rescuing a casualty from a fume-filled environment where there is no fire (for example, a garage), you should first open the doors wide to let in fresh air.

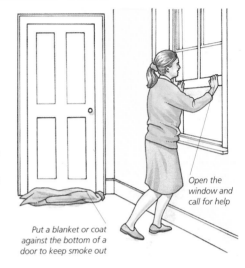

Open the window and call for help

Put a blanket or coat against the bottom of a door to keep smoke out

CLOTHING ON FIRE

The casualty must be prevented from panicking and rushing outside; any movement or breeze will fan the flames.

● Quickly lay the casualty down with the burning side uppermost, and extinguish the flames by dousing the victim with water, or other non-flammable liquid.

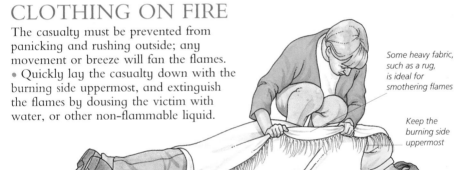

Some heavy fabric, such as a rug, is ideal for smothering flames

Keep the burning side uppermost

● Alternatively, wrap the casualty tightly in a coat, curtain, blanket (not the nylon or cellular type), rug, or other heavy fabric, then lay him on the ground. This starves the flames of oxygen (air), and puts them out.

> DO NOT use flammable materials to try to smother flames.

> DO NOT roll the casualty along the ground. This can cause burning to spread to undamaged parts of the body, and cause other injuries.

IF your own clothes catch fire and help is not available, extinguish the flames by wrapping yourself up tightly in suitable material, and lying down.

21

ELECTRICAL INJURIES

The passage of electrical current through the body may stun the casualty, and cause breathing and even the heart to stop. The current may cause burns both where it enters the body and where it leaves the body to "earth". Alternating current additionally causes muscle spasms that often prevent the casualty from letting go of an electric cable.

Lightning

This is a natural burst of electricity that seeks contact with the ground through the nearest tall feature in the landscape, and, possibly, anyone standing by it. A lightning strike may set clothing on fire and knock the casualty down. Rarely, it may cause instant death. Get away from the site of the strike, and get any casualties away, as soon as possible.

HIGH-VOLTAGE CURRENT

Contact with high-voltage current, found in power lines and overhead high-tension (HT) cables, is usually immediately fatal. Severe burns always result, and the sudden muscular spasm produced by the shock may propel the casualty some distance from the point of contact, causing other injuries, such as fractures.

High-voltage electricity may jump ("arc") up to 18 metres (20 yards). Materials such as dry wood or clothing will not protect you from high-voltage electricity. The power must be cut off *and isolated* before the casualty is approached. This is especially important where railway overhead power lines are damaged.

ACTION

DO NOT approach the casualty until you are officially told that the power has been cut off and, if necessary, isolated. Maintain a distance of at least 18 metres (20 yards) and keep bystanders away.

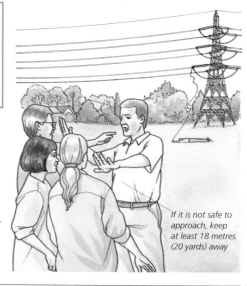

If it is not safe to approach, keep at least 18 metres (20 yards) away

1 Call the emergency services immediately.

2 The casualty will almost certainly be unconscious; once it is safe to do so, check breathing and pulse, and be prepared to resuscitate if necessary. Place him in the recovery position (*see page 30*).

3 Treat any burns (*see page 109*) and associated injuries. Take steps to minimise shock (*see page 68*).

LOW-VOLTAGE CURRENT

Domestic current, as used in homes, offices, workshops, and shops, can cause serious injury, and even death. Many injuries result from faulty switches, frayed flex, or defects within an appliance itself. Young children are especially at risk.

You must be aware of the hazards of water, which is a dangerously good conductor of electricity. Handling an otherwise safe appliance with wet hands, or when standing on a wet floor, substantially increases the risk of a shock.

ACTION

1 Break the contact by switching off the current, at the mains or meter if it can be reached easily. Otherwise, remove the plug, or wrench the cable free.

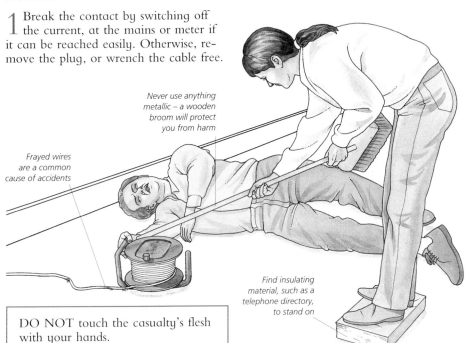

Never use anything metallic – a wooden broom will protect you from harm

Frayed wires are a common cause of accidents

Find insulating material, such as a telephone directory, to stand on

DO NOT touch the casualty's flesh with your hands.

2 If you are unable to reach the cable, socket, or mains:
* Stand on dry insulating material such as a wooden box, a rubber or plastic mat, or thick pile of newspapers. Use a broom, wooden chair or stool to push the casualty's limbs away from the source.
* Without touching the casualty, loop rope around his feet or under the arms and pull him away from the source.
* *As a last resort only,* tug at the casualty's loose, dry clothing.

Once the contact is broken:

IF the casualty is unconscious, check breathing and pulse, and be prepared to resuscitate if necessary. Cool any burns with plenty of cold water (*see page 106*). Place him in the recovery position (*see page 30*), and dial 999 for an ambulance.

IF the casualty seems to be unharmed, he may still be shaken and should be advised to rest. Observe his condition closely and, if in doubt, call a doctor.

RESCUE FROM DROWNING

Open water in and around Britain is cold, even in summer. Sea temperatures range from 5°C (41°F) to 15°C (59°F); inland waters may be even colder. The cold increases the dangers for both casualty and rescuer, as it may cause:
* Uncontrollable gasping on entering the water, with the risk of water inhalation.

* A sudden rise in blood pressure, which can precipitate a heart attack.
* Sudden inability to swim; even a strong swimmer may sink.
* If immersion is prolonged, hypothermia.

See also: Drowning, *page 58.*
          Hypothermia, *page 130.*

ACTION

> YOUR AIM IS:
> * To get the casualty on to dry land with minimum danger to yourself.

Make sure you keep your balance, or the casualty may pull you in

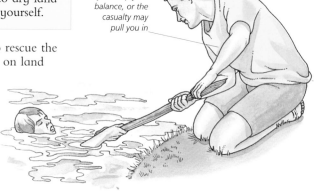

1 Choose the safest way to rescue the casualty. If possible, stay on land and reach with your hand, a stick, or a branch, or throw a rope or float.

> DO NOT enter the water unless it is absolutely necessary.

Support him at the chest to keep it higher than the head

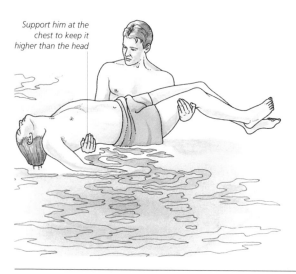

2 Swim to the casualty and tow him only if you are a trained life-saver, or if the casualty is unconscious. It is safer to wade, if you can, than to swim.

3 When bringing the casualty out of the water, carry him with his head lower than his chest, to minimise the dangers of vomiting.

4 Treat for drowning and the effects of cold (*see page 58*).

5 Take or send the casualty to hospital, even if he seems to have recovered well.

RESUSCITATION

It is essential to life that oxygen and other substances taken into the body are transferred, via the bloodstream, to our cells. There, they are converted into the energy required for all the vital processes. The brain, which controls all bodily functions, must have a constant oxygen supply. After three to four minutes' deprivation, brain function begins to fail: consciousness will be lost, breathing and the heartbeat will cease, and death may result.

The ABC of life

Three elements are involved in getting oxygen to the brain. The air passage, or *Airway*, must be open so that oxygen can enter the body; *Breathing* must take place so that oxygen can enter the bloodstream in the lungs; and the blood must travel around the body (the *Circulation*), taking the oxygen to all the tissues, including those of the brain.

What you will find in this chapter

The processes of breathing and circulation, and conditions that affect them, are described in more detail in later chapters. This chapter tells you what you can do to assist a casualty whose breathing and/or heart has stopped. The techniques used to sustain life in the absence of spontaneous breathing and a heartbeat are known as *CardioPulmonary Resuscitation* (*CPR* for short).

THE FIRST AIDER SHOULD:

- Keep the brain supplied with oxygen following the ABC of resuscitation: opening the *Airway*, and maintaining *Breathing* and *Circulation*.

- Get professional help urgently.

CONTENTS

THE PRINCIPLES OF RESUSCITATION

For life to be sustained, a constant supply of oxygen to the brain must be maintained. The oxygen is delivered to its tissues by the circulating blood. The "pump" that maintains this supply is the heart. If the heart stops ("cardiac arrest"), death will result unless urgent action is taken.

In certain circumstances, the use of a machine called a "defibrillator" (*see page 74*), carried in many ambulances, can restart the heart. The casualty is most likely to survive if three needs are met:
• The flow of oxygenated blood is rapidly restored to the brain by means of artificial ventilation and chest compression (cardio-pulmonary resuscitation, or CPR).
• Defibrillation is carried out promptly.
• The casualty quickly reaches hospital to receive specialised treatment and care.

The prompt application of cardio-pulmonary resuscitation may bridge the gap between a casualty's collapse, and the arrival of an ambulancè equipped with a defibrillator. The way in which CPR is performed always follows the same rules – the ABC of resuscitation (*see below*).

Cardiac arrest – the chain of survival
The casualty's chances of survival are greatest when all the links of the chain are in place.

Early access – help is immediately summoned so that a defibrillator can be brought to the casualty.

Early CPR – the techniques of resuscitation are used to buy time until help arrives.

Early defibrillation – a controlled electric shock is given to restart the heart.

Early advanced care – specialised treatment stabilises the casualty's condition.

THE ABC OF RESUSCITATION

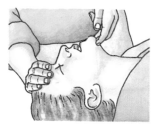

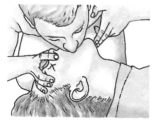

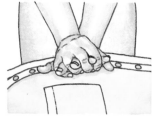

A is for AIRWAY
Tilting the casualty's head back and lifting the chin will "open the airway" – the tilted position lifts the casualty's tongue from the back of the throat so that it does not block the air passage.
See pages 28-29.

B is for BREATHING
If a casualty is not breathing, you can breathe for him or her, and thus oxygenate the blood, by giving "artificial venti-lation" – blowing your own expelled air into the casualty's lungs.
See page 32.

C is for CIRCULATION
If the heart has stopped, "chest compressions" can be applied to force blood through the heart and around the body. They must be combined with artificial ventilation so that the blood is oxygenated.
See page 34.

ASSESSING THE CASUALTY

A quick assessment of a collapsed casualty will indicate the most urgent priority and dictate your action. The charts below show you how to use this assessment to make an instant, and possibly life-saving, decision about the course of action you should take.

The upper chart tells you what steps to take to assess the situation, and the casualty's condition. For guidance on dealing with danger, turn to the chapter *Action at an Emergency (pages 13-24)*. Step-by-step guides to assessing the casualty are given overleaf.

The lower chart tells you how best to act on your findings. For example, in the worst possible situation, your assessment will have told you that an unconscious casualty is not breathing, nor does he or she have a pulse (the casualty will be in "cardiac arrest").

The chart shows you that in this situation, the sequence of action that will give the casualty the greatest chance of survival is to first telephone for an ambulance, or get someone else to do so, then start and continue artificial ventilation and chest compression.

ASSESS THE CASUALTY'S CONDITION

Danger	Are you or the casualty in any danger?
Response	Is the casualty conscious?
Airway	Is the airway open and clear?
Breathing	Is the casualty breathing?
Circulation	Is there a pulse?

ACT ON YOUR FINDINGS

Unconscious, no pulse or breathing	1 Dial 999 for an ambulance. 2 Start and continue artificial ventilation and chest compression.
Unconscious, no breathing, pulse present	1 Give 10 breaths of artificial ventilation. 2 Dial 999 for an ambulance. 3 Continue artificial ventilation.
Unconscious, breathing and pulse present	1 Treat any life-threatening injury. 2 Place the casualty in the recovery position. 3 Get help.
Conscious, breathing and pulse present	1 Treat as appropriate. 2 Get help if necessary.

MAKING YOUR ASSESSMENT

You may see someone collapse in front of you. More commonly, you will come across, or be called to help, someone who has already collapsed. In every case you should rapidly carry out a brief assessment (preferably without moving the casualty), following the ABC of resuscitation, in order to determine your priorities and actions. Your assessment will answer three vital questions:
• Is the casualty conscious?
• Is the casualty breathing?
• Is there a pulse?

CHECK FOR CONSCIOUSNESS

Ask a question or give a command – for example, "What's happened?" or "Open your eyes!" – speaking loudly and clearly, close to the casualty's ear. Carefully shake the casualty's shoulders.
• A casualty in a serious state of "altered consciousness" may mumble, groan, or make slight movements.
• A fully unconscious casualty will not respond.

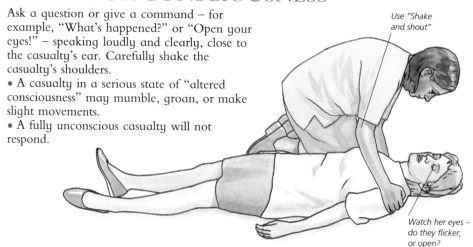

Use "Shake and shout"

Watch her eyes – do they flicker, or open?

OPEN THE AIRWAY

An unconscious casualty's airway may be narrowed or blocked, making breathing difficult and noisy, or impossible.

The main reason for this is that muscular control in the throat is lost, which allows the tongue to sag back and block the throat. Lifting the chin and tilting the head back lifts the tongue away from the entrance to the air passage.

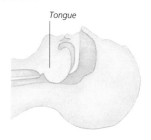

Tongue

Blocked airway
Unconsciousness disables the muscles, allowing the tongue to sag and block the throat. The casualty cannot breathe.

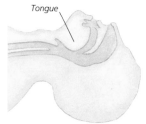

Tongue

Open airway
"Head tilt and chin lift" positions the head so that the tongue is lifted from the back of the throat, leaving the airway clear.

TO OPEN THE AIRWAY

1 Remove any obvious obstruction from the mouth.

2 Placing two fingers under the point of the casualty's chin, lift the jaw. At the same time, place your other hand on the casualty's forehead, and tilt the head well back.

IF you suspect head or neck injuries, handle the head carefully, tilting it only just far enough to open the airway.

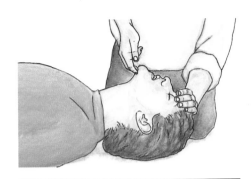

CHECK FOR BREATHING

Put your face close to the casualty's mouth, and look, listen, and feel for breathing:
• *Look* for chest movements.
• *Listen* for sounds of breathing.
• *Feel* for breath on your cheek.
Look, listen, and feel for five seconds before deciding that breathing is absent.

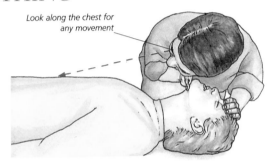

Look along the chest for any movement

CHECK FOR A PULSE

If the heart is beating adequately it will generate a pulse in the neck (the *carotid* pulse) where the main carotid arteries pass up to the head. These arteries lie on either side of the larynx, between the Adam's apple and the "strap muscle" that runs from behind the ear across the neck to the top of the breastbone.

TO CHECK THE CAROTID PULSE

1 With the head tilted back, feel for the Adam's apple with two fingers. Slide your fingers back towards you into the gap between the Adam's apple and the strap muscle, and feel for the carotid pulse.

2 Feel for five seconds before deciding that the pulse is absent.

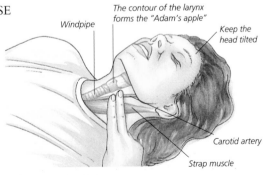

Windpipe

The contour of the larynx forms the "Adam's apple"

Keep the head tilted

Carotid artery

Strap muscle

29

THE RECOVERY POSITION

Any unconscious casualty should be placed in the recovery position. This position prevents the tongue from blocking the throat, and, because the head is slightly lower than the rest of the body, it allows liquids to drain from the mouth, reducing the risk of the casualty inhaling stomach contents. The head, neck, and back are kept in a straight line, while the bent limbs keep the body propped in a secure and comfortable position. If you must leave an unconscious casualty unattended, he or she can safely be left in the recovery position while you get help.

The technique for turning shown below assumes that the casualty is lying on her back from the start. Not all the steps will be necessary if a casualty is found lying on his or her side or front.

Before turning a casualty, remove his or her spectacles, if worn, and any bulky objects from pockets.

METHOD

1 Kneeling beside the casualty, open her airway by tilting the head and lifting the chin. Straighten her legs. Place the arm nearest you out at right-angles to her body, elbow bent, and with the hand palm uppermost.

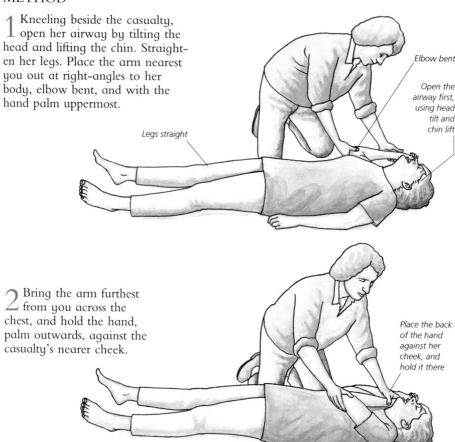

Legs straight

Elbow bent

Open the airway first, using head tilt and chin lift

2 Bring the arm furthest from you across the chest, and hold the hand, palm outwards, against the casualty's nearer cheek.

Place the back of the hand against her cheek, and hold it there

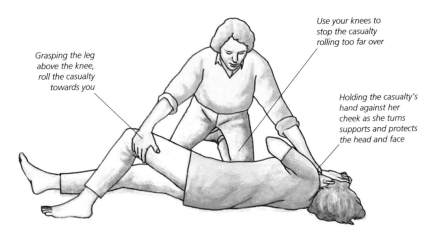

Grasping the leg above the knee, roll the casualty towards you

Use your knees to stop the casualty rolling too far over

Holding the casualty's hand against her cheek as she turns supports and protects the head and face

3 With your other hand, grasp the thigh furthest from you and pull the knee up, keeping the foot flat on the ground.

4 Keeping her hand pressed against her cheek, pull at the thigh to roll the casualty towards you and on to her side.

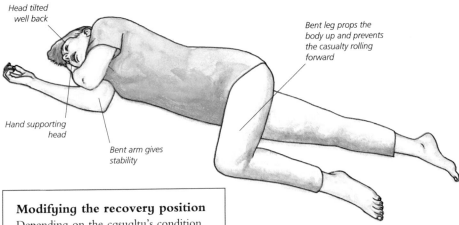

Head tilted well back

Bent leg props the body up and prevents the casualty rolling forward

Hand supporting head

Bent arm gives stability

Modifying the recovery position

Depending on the casualty's condition, you may have to modify the recovery position to avoid making injuries worse. For example, an unconscious casualty with a spinal injury needs extra support at the head and neck during turning, and in the final position, to keep the head and trunk aligned at all times (*see* page 157). If limbs are injured and cannot be bent, use extra helpers or place rolled blankets against the casualty's body to prevent it toppling forward.

5 Tilt the head back to make sure the airway remains open. Adjust the hand under the cheek, if necessary, so that the head stays in this tilted position.

6 Adjust the upper leg, if necessary, so that both the hip and the knee are bent at right-angles.

7 Dial 999 for an ambulance. Check breathing and pulse frequently while waiting for help to arrive.

ARTIFICIAL VENTILATION

Expired air still contains 16 per cent oxygen, so you can use it to "breathe" for a casualty by blowing it into his or her lungs. The way this is done depends on the casualty's condition:
• If a casualty has stopped breathing but still has a pulse, give 10 breaths of artificial ventilation, telephone for help, then continue at a rate of 10 breaths per minute until the casualty starts to breathe on his or her own, or until help arrives. Check for a pulse after every 10 breaths.
• If the casualty's breathing *and* pulse have stopped, you must first phone for

help, then combine artificial ventilation with chest compression (*see page 34*). *The Sequence of CPR*, on page 38, explains how this is done.

Using face shields

Artificial ventilation carries little or no risk of the transfer of infection. However, for hygienic purposes, regular First Aiders may be trained in the use of disposable plastic face shields. If you are trained to use a shield, carry one at all times – but if you do not have one with you, you should *never* hesitate to give artificial ventilation.

MOUTH-TO-MOUTH VENTILATION

1 With the casualty lying flat on his back, first remove any obvious obstruction, including broken or displaced dentures, from the mouth. Leave well-fitting dentures in place.

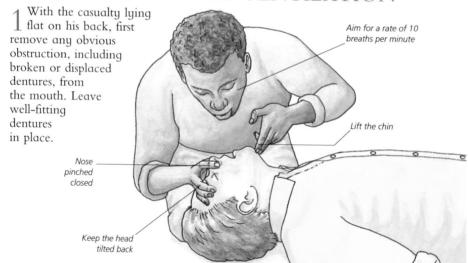

Aim for a rate of 10 breaths per minute

Lift the chin

Nose pinched closed

Keep the head tilted back

2 Open the airway by tilting the head and lifting the chin (*see page 29*).

3 Close the casualty's nose by pinching it with your index finger and thumb. Take a full breath, and place your lips around his mouth, making a good seal.

4 Blow into the casualty's mouth until you see the chest rise. Take about two seconds for full inflation.

5 Remove your lips and allow the chest to fall fully. Deliver subsequent breaths in the same manner.

IF THE CHEST DOES NOT RISE

If you cannot get breaths into the casualty's chest, check that:
- The head is tilted sufficiently far back.
- You have a firm seal around the casualty's mouth.
- You have closed the nostrils completely.
- The airway is not obstructed by vomit, blood or a foreign body.

CLEARING AN OBSTRUCTION

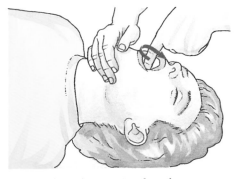

1 Providing the jaw is relaxed, sweep a finger around inside the mouth. Be very careful to avoid the back of the throat if doing this to a young child.

2 If this fails, give backslaps and abdominal thrusts (*see page 57*).

Other forms of artificial ventilation

In situations such as rescue from water, or where mouth injuries make a good seal impossible, you may choose to use the mouth-to-nose method of artificial ventilation. While it is usually easy to blow air into the nose, it is not so easy for the air to escape; the soft parts of the nose may flop back like a valve.

To give mouth-to-nose ventilation
1 With the casualty's mouth closed, form a tight seal with your lips around the casualty's nose, and blow.
2 Open the mouth to let the breath out. Continue at the normal rate.
  Babies should be given artificial ventilation using the mouth-to-mouth-and-nose method (*see page 37*).

Mouth-to-stoma ventilation
A laryngectomee is someone whose voice box (*larynx*) has been surgically removed, leaving a permanent opening (*stoma*) in the front of the neck through which breathing takes place.
  Artificial ventilation must be given through the stoma. If the chest fails to rise and your air escapes from the casualty's mouth, he or she may be a "partial neck breather"; you will have to close off the mouth and nose with your thumb and fingers while giving mouth-to-stoma ventilation.

DO NOT use any form of abdominal thrust on babies.

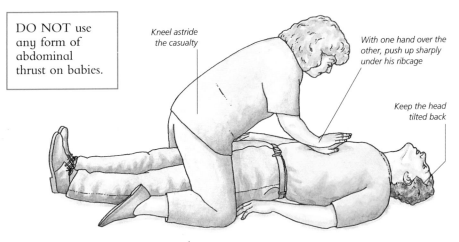

Kneel astride the casualty

With one hand over the other, push up sharply under his ribcage

Keep the head tilted back

RESTORING THE CIRCULATION

If there is no pulse, the heart has stopped. You will have to provide an artificial circulation by performing chest compressions, which will send blood to the brain. To be of any use to the brain, this supply of blood must be oxygenated, therefore chest compression must be combined with artificial ventilation in the way laid out in *The Sequence of CPR*, on page 38.

CHEST COMPRESSION

1 With the casualty lying flat on his back on a firm surface, kneel beside him, and find one of his lowest ribs using your index and middle fingers. Slide your fingers upwards to the point in the middle where the rib margins meet at the breastbone. Place your middle finger over this point (the *xiphisternum*) and your index finger on the breastbone (*sternum*) above.

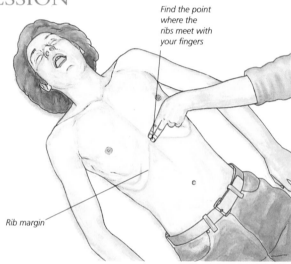

Find the point where the ribs meet with your fingers

Rib margin

2 Place the heel of your other hand on the breastbone, and slide it down until it reaches your index finger. This is the point at which you will apply pressure.

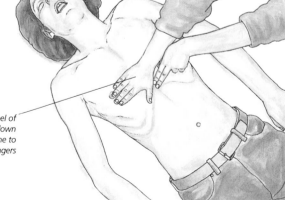

Slide the heel of your hand down the breastbone to meet the fingers

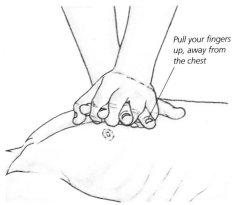

Pull your fingers up, away from the chest

3 Place the heel of your first hand on top of the other hand, and interlock the fingers.

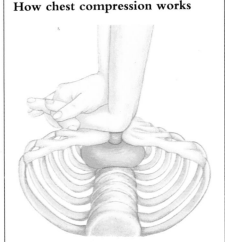

How chest compression works

Pushing down on the breastbone causes pressure changes within the chest that expel blood from the heart's chambers, forcing it towards the tissues. As the pressure is released, the chest rises, and replacement blood is "sucked" in to refill the heart; this blood is then forced out of the heart by the next compression.

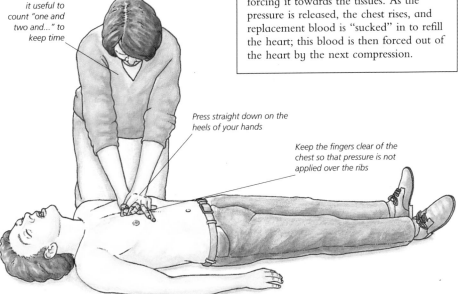

You may find it useful to count "one and two and..." to keep time

Press straight down on the heels of your hands

Keep the fingers clear of the chest so that pressure is not applied over the ribs

4 Leaning well over the casualty, with your arms straight, press down vertically on the breastbone to depress it approximately 4-5cm (1½-2in), then release the pressure without removing your hands.

5 Repeat the compressions, aiming for a rate of approximately 80 compressions per minute. To combine with artificial ventilation, follow the sequence shown on page 38.

RESUSCITATION FOR CHILDREN

It is rare for a child's heart to stop but there are dangers in airway blockage. The main difference in approach is the need to give artificial ventilation for one minute before calling an ambulance. Artificial ventilation and chest compression can be performed on older children just as for adults, but slightly faster and with lighter pressure. The technique requires some modifications for small children and babies.

CHECKING FOR A BABY'S BREATHING

Open the airway by gently lifting the chin and tilting the head slightly. Look, listen, and feel for breathing.

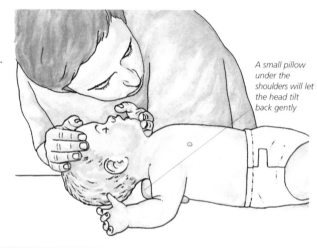

A small pillow under the shoulders will let the head tilt back gently

DO NOT, if clearing an obstruction with a finger, touch the back of a young child's throat. If the child is suffering from an in-fection of the airway, this can cause swelling and, possibly, total blockage (*see page 64*).

CHECKING FOR A BABY'S CIRCULATION

It is difficult to feel the carotid pulse in an infant so, instead, use the *brachial* pulse. This is located on the inside of the upper arm, midway between shoulder and elbow.

    Place your index and middle fingers on the inside of the arm, and press lightly towards the bone. It may help to place your thumb on the outside of the arm. Feel for 5 seconds before deciding there is no pulse.

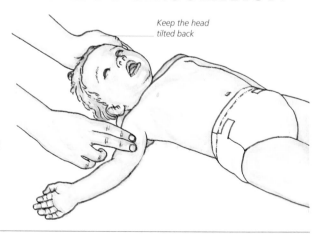

Keep the head tilted back

ARTIFICIAL VENTILATION FOR A BABY

Give artificial ventilation to babies, with mouth-to-mouth-and-nose technique, at twice the rate for adults. Seal around the baby's mouth and nose with your mouth, then breathe into the lungs until the chest rises. Let it fall.

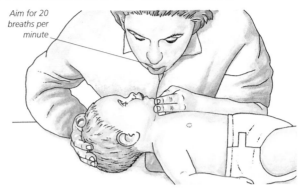

Aim for 20 breaths per minute

Give five breaths, then check the pulse. If the pulse is present and adequate but breathing is absent, continue at a rate of 20 breaths per minute.

CHEST COMPRESSION

If you cannot detect a pulse, apply chest compressions to the lower half of the breastbone. Use the adult technique for an older child; for babies and small children, modify the technique and rate as below. Remember that, in the absence of a pulse, chest compression must be combined with artificial ventilation.

FOR A BABY

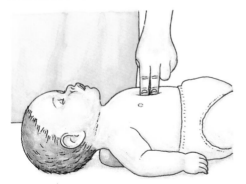

Lay the baby on a firm surface. To locate the correct position, imagine a line joining the baby's nipples. Place the tips of two fingers just below the mid-point of this line, and press at a rate of 100 compressions per minute, to a depth of 1.5–2.5cm (½–1in).

Combine with artificial ventilation, giving five compressions to one breath.

FOR A SMALL CHILD

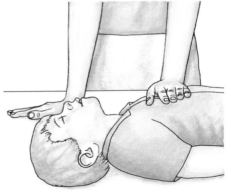

Find the correct position on the chest as you would for an adult (*see page 34*). Using one hand only, press at a rate of 100 compressions per minute, depressing the chest by 2.5–3cm (1–1½in).

Combine with artificial ventilation, giving five compressions to one breath.

THE SEQUENCE OF CPR

When a casualty has no pulse and is not breathing, you must combine artificial ventilation with chest compression. This is the sequence known as CPR (cardiopulmonary resuscitation).

If you are alone with an adult casualty, you must if possible call for help before you start CPR. With a baby or child, give CPR for a full minute before calling an ambulance. Once you have started, continue resuscitation until professional help arrives, the pulse and breathing return, or exhaustion forces you to stop.

See also: Artificial ventilation, *page 32.*
Chest compression, *page 34.*

FOR ONE FIRST AIDER

1 Immediately dial 999 for an ambulance.
2 Open the casualty's airway by tilting the head and lifting the chin, and give two breaths of artificial ventilation. Don't wait for the chest to deflate after the second breath.
3 Move your hands to the casualty's chest, and give 15 chest compressions.
4 Return to the head and give two more ventilations, then 15 further compressions.
5 Continue to give two ventilations every 15 compressions until help arrives.

It is very unlikely that you will be rewarded by the heart re-starting before expert assistance is given. Do not interrupt CPR to make pulse checks unless there is any sign of a returning circulation. With a pulse confirmed, check breathing and, if it is still absent, continue with artificial ventilation. Check the pulse after every 10 breaths, and be prepared to re-start chest compressions if it disappears. If the casualty starts to breathe unaided, place him or her in the recovery position. Re-check breathing and pulse every two minutes.

FOR TWO FIRST AIDERS

One person should go to summon help while the other immediately starts CPR.

Then, either proceed as above, each person taking it in turn, or, while one of you gives chest compressions, the other can give one breath of artificial ventilation after every *five* compressions. Pause to ensure that the casualty's chest rises, but *do not wait* for the chest to fall before continuing with chest compression.

In practice, it is easier to work on the opposite side of the casualty to your partner

Rest while your partner delivers a breath

Give one breath after every five compressions

THE PRACTICE OF FIRST AID

When giving first aid treatment to any casualty it is important to work to a plan. "First Aiders" are trained in routines that can be applied to many situations. The initial priorities – ensuring safety, and following the ABC of resuscitation – have been covered in the previous two chapters. Only when the casualty is out of danger can you begin to treat illness or injury.

Diagnosis and treatment

In most situations that require first aid, there will be no life-threatening danger. You will simply be assisting a conscious casualty, whose recovery from some minor injury or illness is not in doubt. However, in every case, your aim is to discover what is wrong with the casualty, and to give prompt, correct treatment in a logical order. This chapter will help you to carry out these tasks.

CONTENTS

THE FIRST AIDER SHOULD:

Preserve life
- Pay strict attention to safety (*pages 13-24*).
- Follow the ABC of resuscitation (*pages 25-38*).
- Look for and control any major bleeding (*page 78*).

Limit the effects of the condition
- Make a diagnosis of the illness or injury, if possible, by means of a thorough examination.
- Treat casualties in a sensible order of priority.
- Treat multiple injuries in a sensible order of priority. Remember the possibility of "hidden" secondary illnesses or conditions.

Promote the casualty's recovery
- Relieve any anxiety, pain, and discomfort.
- Arrange for appropriate medical attention.

MAKING A DIAGNOSIS

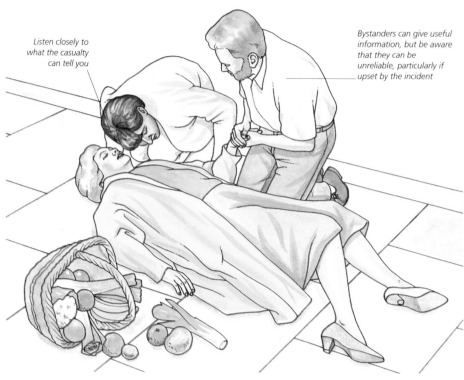

Listen closely to what the casualty can tell you

Bystanders can give useful information, but be aware that they can be unreliable, particularly if upset by the incident

Once it is safe to start giving treatment, you must first identify what is wrong with the casualty. The process by which you recognise what is wrong is called *diagnosis*; this will often involve suspicion rather than certainty. Your diagnosis will be a conclusion, based upon a high degree of reasonable probability, on which you should be prepared to act.

Making a diagnosis often requires a thorough physical examination (*see page 44*). Factors that will help you include history and clues to any medical condition (*see opposite*), and symptoms and signs (*see overleaf*). Throughout this book, the probable history, symptoms, and signs of specific illnesses and injuries are grouped under the heading *Recognition*.

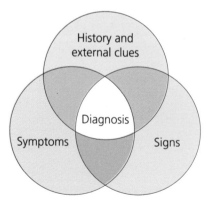

Aids to diagnosis
The diagnosis you make will be a conclusion based on reasonable probability. You will reach such a conclusion using information from many sources, which can be grouped in three categories – history and clues, symptoms, and signs.

HISTORY

This is the full story of how the incident occurred, how the injury was sustained, or how the illness began. It should include anything you can discover about past illness or injury, and should be obtained directly from the casualty. If he or she is unconscious, question onlookers.

Picture what happened

In cases of injury, try to form a complete picture of what took place. Try to assess the amount of force involved, and how it was applied to cause injury.

• Consider the casualty's age and state of health. For example, a young, fit adult who trips over a kerb may sprain a wrist, whereas a frail elderly lady who does the same is more likely to break her arm, and possibly also her hip.
• Always ask whether the casualty is suffering from any illness and/or is taking any medicines.
• Try to establish who the casualty is, and where he or she lives.
• Make a note of all relevant information so that you can pass it on.

EXTERNAL CLUES

If the casualty is unconscious or uncooperative, look through pockets and bags for clues (beware of syringes if you suspect drug abuse). There may be an appointment card for a hospital or clinic, or a special card that tells you that the casualty is on medication, or gives other medical details (for example, a history of allergy or epilepsy). Horse-riders may carry such a card in their riding hat.

Medication carried by the casualty may give valuable pointers to the cause of the emergency. Medical warning items ("Medic-Alert", "SOS Talisman") may be worn as a medallion, bracelet, or locket, or on a key ring. Some of these devices contain a piece of paper giving medical information. If you find one of these, take great care not to lose or damage it, and return it to the casualty.

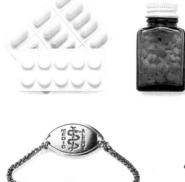

Medicines
Glyceryl trinitrate is taken for angina, for example; *phenobarbitone* or *phenytoin* for epilepsy. Simpler remedies may give clues – indigestion tablets could indicate a stomach ulcer.

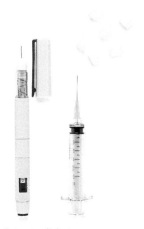

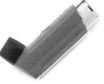

Pointers to diabetes
An insulin syringe (which may look like a pen) and/or sugar lumps tell you that the casualty is a diabetic.

Warning bracelet
This example gives a telephone number for information about the casualty's medical history.

Inhaler
"Puffer" aerosol inhalers like the one shown here are frequently carried by asthmatics.

SYMPTOMS AND SIGNS

Every injury and illness manifests itself in distinctive ways that may help your diagnosis. These clues are divided into two groups: *symptoms* and *signs*. Some will be obvious, but other valuable ones may be overlooked unless you examine the casualty thoroughly from head to toe (*see* *overleaf*). A conscious casualty should be examined, wherever possible, in the position found, or with any obvious injury comfortably supported; an unconscious casualty's airway must first be opened and secured.

Use your senses – look, listen, feel, and smell. Be quick and alert, but be thorough, and do not skimp or make assumptions. Ask the casualty to describe any sensations your touch causes as the examination proceeds. Though you should handle the casualty gently, your touch must be firm enough to ensure that you will feel any swelling or irregularity, or detect a tender spot.

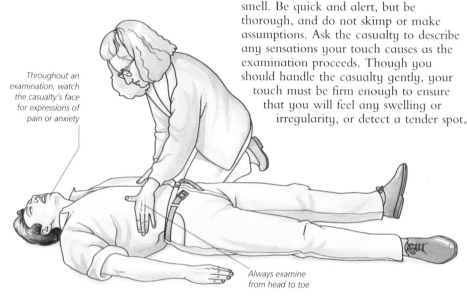

Throughout an examination, watch the casualty's face for expressions of pain or anxiety

Always examine from head to toe

CHECKING FOR SYMPTOMS

These are sensations that the casualty feels or experiences, and may be able to describe. You may need to ask questions to establish their presence or absence. Ask a conscious casualty if there is any pain and exactly where it is felt. Examine that part particularly, and then any other sites where pain is felt; severe pain in one place can mask a more serious, but less painful injury at another.

Other symptoms that may help you include nausea, giddiness, heat, cold, weakness, and impaired sensation. All symptoms should be assessed and confirmed, wherever appropriate, by an examination for signs of injury or illness.

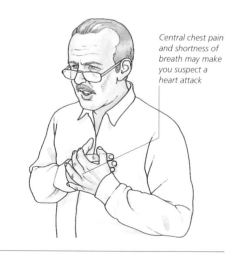

Central chest pain and shortness of breath may make you suspect a heart attack

LOOKING FOR SIGNS

These are details discovered by applying your senses – sight, touch, hearing, and smell – often in the course of an examination. Common signs of injury include bleeding, swelling, tenderness, or deformity; signs of illness that are very often evident are a pale or flushed skin, sweating, a raised body temperature, and a rapid pulse.

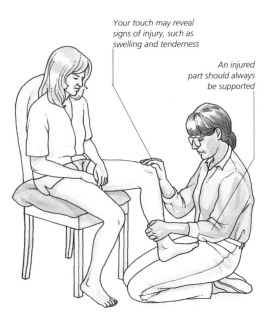

Your touch may reveal signs of injury, such as swelling and tenderness

An injured part should always be supported

Making a diagnosis from signs

Many signs are immediately obvious, but others may be discovered only in the course of thorough physical examination (*see overleaf*). If the casualty is unconscious, confused or otherwise unreliable, your diagnosis may have to be formed purely on the basis of the circumstances of the incident, information obtained from onlookers, and the signs you discover.

SYMPTOMS AND SIGNS OF INJURY OR ILLNESS

The casualty may tell you of these *symptoms*	Pain • Apprehension • Heat • Cold • Loss of normal movement • Loss of sensation • Abnormal sensation • Thirst • Nausea • Tingling • Faintness • Stiffness • Momentary unconsciousness • Weakness • Memory loss • Dizziness • Sensation of broken bone
You may see these *signs*	Anxiety and painful expression • Unusual chest movement • Sweating • Wounds • Bleeding from orifices • Response to touch • Response to speech • Bruising • Abnormal skin colour • Muscle spasm • Swelling • Deformity • Foreign bodies • Needle marks • Vomit • Incontinence • Containers and other circumstantial evidence
Your sense of touch may reveal these *signs*	Dampness • Abnormal body temperature • Tenderness to touch or pressure • Swelling • Deformity • Irregularity • Grating bone ends
You may hear these *signs*	Noisy or distressed breathing • Groaning • Sucking sounds (chest injury) • Response to touch • Response to speech
Your sense of smell may detect these *signs*. Remember to smell the casualty's breath	Acetone • Alcoholic liquors • Burning • Gas or fumes • Solvents or glue • Incontinence

TOP-TO-TOE SURVEY

Having taken any life-saving action, carefully examine the casualty. Start always at the head and work down; the "top-to-toe" routine is both easily remembered and thorough. You may need to move or remove clothing (see page 46), but bear in mind that, during every stage of your examination, you should try not to move the casualty more than is absolutely necessary.

Use both hands, and always compare one side of the body with the other, since any swelling or deformity may be revealed much more clearly.

Skull and scalp

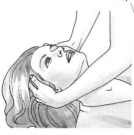

Run your hands over the scalp to find bleeding, swelling, or any soft area or indentation that might indicate a fracture. Handle the head and neck very gently.

Nose

Check for any sign of blood or clear fluid (or a mixture of both) that might indicate damage inside the skull.

Face

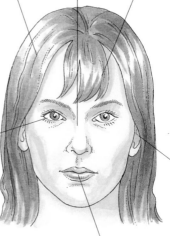

Note the colour, the temperature, and the state of the skin. For example, the closed eyes, open mouth, and noisy breathing of unconsciousness may be accompanied by the pale, cold, sweaty skin that indicates shock, or the flushed, hot face of heatstroke or fever.

Eyes

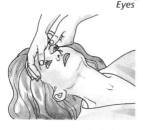

Examine both eyes together, noting the size of the dark circular centres (the pupils), and whether they are equal in size. Look for any foreign body, wound, or bruising in the whites of the eyes.

Ears

Speak to the casualty. Ask if she can hear in both ears. Look for blood or clear fluid (or a mixture of both) coming from either ear canal that might indicate damage inside the skull.

Mouth

Record the rate, depth, and nature (easy or difficult, noisy or quiet) of breathing. Note any odour on the breath. Look and feel inside the mouth for anything that might endanger the airway. If dentures are intact and fit firmly, leave them in place. Look for any wound in the mouth or irregularity in the line of the teeth. Examine the lips for burns or discoloration, particularly blueness (which indicates low blood oxygen).

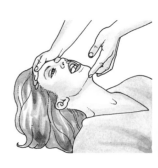

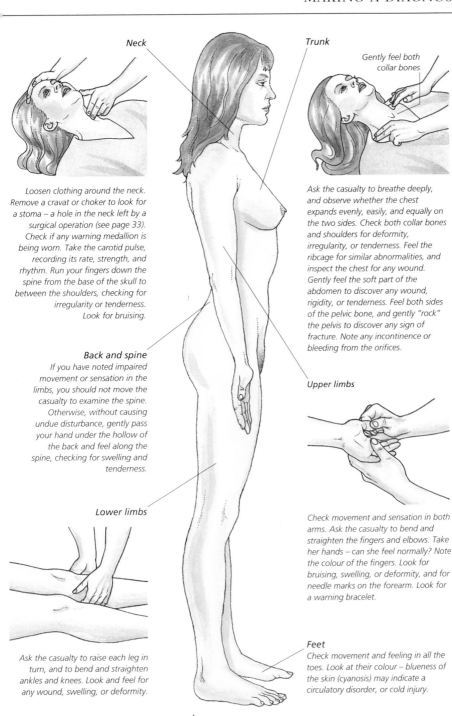

Neck

Loosen clothing around the neck. Remove a cravat or choker to look for a stoma – a hole in the neck left by a surgical operation (see page 33). Check if any warning medallion is being worn. Take the carotid pulse, recording its rate, strength, and rhythm. Run your fingers down the spine from the base of the skull to between the shoulders, checking for irregularity or tenderness. Look for bruising.

Back and spine

If you have noted impaired movement or sensation in the limbs, you should not move the casualty to examine the spine. Otherwise, without causing undue disturbance, gently pass your hand under the hollow of the back and feel along the spine, checking for swelling and tenderness.

Lower limbs

Ask the casualty to raise each leg in turn, and to bend and straighten ankles and knees. Look and feel for any wound, swelling, or deformity.

Trunk

Gently feel both collar bones

Ask the casualty to breathe deeply, and observe whether the chest expands evenly, easily, and equally on the two sides. Check both collar bones and shoulders for deformity, irregularity, or tenderness. Feel the ribcage for similar abnormalities, and inspect the chest for any wound. Gently feel the soft part of the abdomen to discover any wound, rigidity, or tenderness. Feel both sides of the pelvic bone, and gently "rock" the pelvis to discover any sign of fracture. Note any incontinence or bleeding from the orifices.

Upper limbs

Check movement and sensation in both arms. Ask the casualty to bend and straighten the fingers and elbows. Take her hands – can she feel normally? Note the colour of the fingers. Look for bruising, swelling, or deformity, and for needle marks on the forearm. Look for a warning bracelet.

Feet

Check movement and feeling in all the toes. Look at their colour – blueness of the skin (cyanosis) may indicate a circulatory disorder, or cold injury.

REMOVING CLOTHING

Sometimes it is necessary to remove clothing in order to expose injuries, make an accurate diagnosis, or conduct a proper treatment. This should be done with the minimum of disturbance to the casualty. Only remove as much as is actually necessary, and try where possible to respect the casualty's feelings and maintain privacy. Do not damage clothing unless it is absolutely necessary, and always, where you can, cut along the seams.

REMOVING SHOES

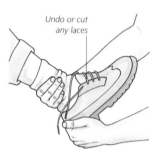

Undo or cut any laces

Support the ankle as you carefully remove the shoe. Long boots with no zip may need to be carefully slit down the back seam with a sharp knife.

REMOVING SOCKS

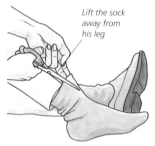

Lift the sock away from his leg

If socks are difficult to pull off, insert two fingers between the sock and the leg. Raise the sock and cut alongside your fingers with scissors.

REMOVING TROUSERS

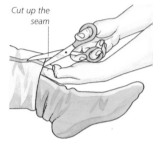

Cut up the seam

Pull them down from the waist to reveal the thigh, or pull up the trouser leg to expose the calf and knee. If necessary, slit up the seam.

REMOVING A COAT OR SHIRT

1 Raise the casualty, and pull the garment off his shoulders.

2 Bend his arm on the uninjured side, and remove the coat from that side first.

3 Then slip the injured arm out of its sleeve, keeping the arm straight if possible.

IF necessary, slit up the sleeve or side seam on the casualty's injured side. Try not to cause too much damage.

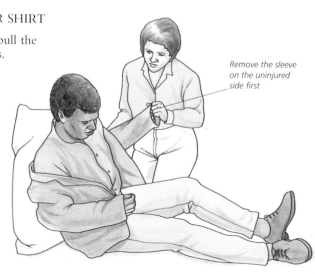

Remove the sleeve on the uninjured side first

REMOVING CRASH-HELMETS

A protective helmet, such as a motorcycle crash-helmet, is best left on, and should only be removed if absolutely necessary (for example, if it prevents you from performing artificial ventilation). Any helmet should always, if possible, be removed by the casualty.

Do not remove a full-face helmet (that encloses the head and face) unless it obstructs breathing, or the casualty is vomiting, or there are severe head injuries. Removal ideally requires two people, so that the casualty's head and neck are constantly supported.

FOR AN OPEN-FACE HELMET OR RIDING HAT

DO NOT remove the helmet unless it is absolutely necessary.

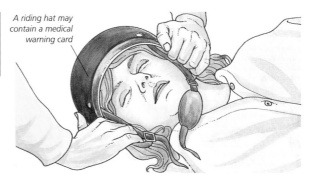

A riding hat may contain a medical warning card

1 Unfasten the buckle, or cut through the chinstrap.

2 Force the helmet's sides apart to take pressure off the head, then lift the helmet upwards and backwards.

FOR A FULL-FACE HELMET

DO NOT remove the helmet unless it is absolutely necessary.

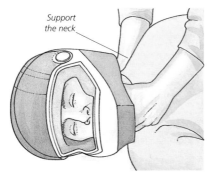

Support the neck

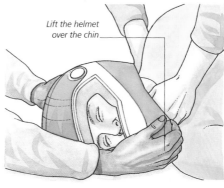

Lift the helmet over the chin

1 Working from the base of the helmet, ease your fingers underneath the rim. Support the neck and hold the lower jaw firmly, with your fingers spread.

2 Ask a helper to tilt the helmet (not the head) back, working from above, and gently lift it until it is clear of the chin.

3 While you continue to support the neck and jaw, your helper should tilt the helmet forwards to pass over the base of the skull, then lift it straight off.

TREATMENT AND AFTERCARE

Calmly and efficiently, treat each condition found. Pay attention to the casualty's remarks or requests. Reassure the casualty constantly, but do not pester him or her with questions.

Establishing treatment priorities

Follow this order as applicable; your own common sense and judgement will dictate modifications.
* Follow the ABC of resuscitation.
* Control bleeding.
* Treat large wounds, burns, and fractures.
* Look for and treat other injuries or conditions.
* Treat for shock.

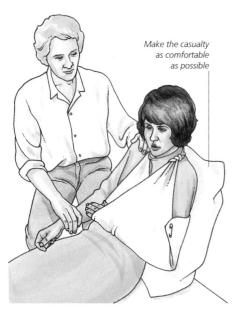

Make the casualty as comfortable as possible

While giving the necessary treatment, help the casualty into a correct and comfortable position. Do not let people crowd around.

Use your judgement to decide whether the casualty needs medical treatment and, if so, what level of attention is required. If you have to summon help, send someone else to do so whenever possible, in case the casualty's condition alters or worsens. Stay with the casualty until the doctor or ambulance arrives.

DO NOT give anything by mouth to a casualty who is unconscious, who may have internal injuries, or who may require hospital treatment.

DO NOT send anyone home who has been unconscious for longer than three minutes, has had severe breathing difficulty, or has displayed the features of shock.

Dealing with the casualty's belongings

If you have to search a casualty's personal belongings, do so only in the presence of a reliable witness. Take care of any property found, and hand it over to the police or ambulance personnel.

Make sure someone accepts responsibility for getting a message to the casualty's home. If involved, the police will do this – if not, volunteer your help.

Arranging for further care

Depending on your assessment of the casualty's condition, you may:
* Dial 999 for an ambulance.
* Arrange transport to hospital by ambulance or other suitable vehicle.
* Hand over the casualty to the care of a doctor, nurse, or ambulance officer.
* Take the casualty to a nearby house or shelter to await medical help.
* Call the casualty's doctor (or any doctor) for advice.
* Allow the casualty to go home, accompanied if possible. Ask the casualty if someone will be at home to meet him or her, or if you can help arrange this. Advise the casualty to see a doctor.

PASSING ON INFORMATION

Having summoned medical aid, make notes, if possible, so that you can pass on all the information you have gathered about the casualty. Always include a record of the casualty's pulse, breathing, and level of response, made at least every 10 minutes for as long as he or she remains in your care. You may wish to check more frequently if the casualty is in a critical condition. The observation chart overleaf, which is recommended for use by all three Voluntary Aid Societies, will enable you to note your findings clearly.

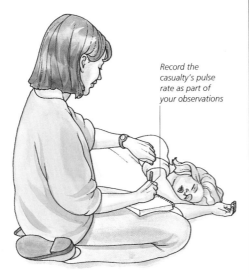

Record the casualty's pulse rate as part of your observations

Make a brief written report to accompany your observations. A record of the timing of events is particularly valuable to medical personnel. Note carefully, for example, the length of a period of unconsciousness, the duration of a fit, the time of any changes in the casualty's condition, and the time of any intervention or treatment.

If possible, stay with the casualty until help arrives, or accompany him or her to hospital, so that you can hand your notes over personally.

Making a report

Your report should include:
- The casualty's name and address.
- History of the accident or illness.
- A brief description of any injuries.
- Any unusual behaviour.
- Any treatment given, and when.
- The following observations, recorded every 10 minutes:

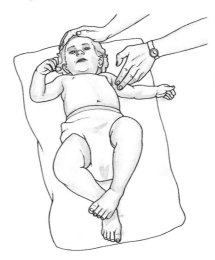

Pulse Take the pulse at the wrist (the *radial* pulse, *page 67*), the neck (the *carotid* pulse, *page 29*), or on a baby's upper arm (the *brachial* pulse, *page 36*). Note the rate over one minute, and whether it is weak or strong, regular or irregular.

Breathing Count the number of times the casualty breathes over one minute, and note whether breathing is quiet and easy, or noisy and difficult.

Level of response Measure and record the responses the casualty makes to certain stimuli in the three categories given on the chart overleaf.

Speak clearly and directly, close to the casualty's ear. Apply a painful stimulus by pinching the skin, or by squeezing the Achilles tendon at the back of the heel.

OBSERVATION CHART

This chart will enable you to make a clear record of your observations (by ticking the appropriate boxes), and update them at intervals while waiting for help to arrive. Always send the completed chart, and any other notes, with the casualty when he or she leaves your care. This information can be very valuable when decisions are taken about further treatment.

CASUALTY'S NAME	DATE							
	Time (10-minute intervals)							
Eyes	Open spontaneously							
	Open to speech							
	Open to painful stimulus							
	No response							
Movement	Obeys commands							
	Responds to painful stimulus							
	No response							
Speech	Normal							
	Confused							
	Uses inappropriate words							
	Incomprehensible							
	No response							
Pulse (beats per minute)	111-120							
	101-110							
	91-100							
	81-90							
	71-80							
	61-70							
	51-60							
Breathing (breaths per minute)	41-50							
	31-40							
	21-30							
	11-20							
	1-10							

DISORDERS OF AIRWAY AND BREATHING

O xygen is essential to support life. The process of breathing enables air containing oxygen to be taken into the lungs, so that the oxygen can be transferred to the blood and circulated throughout the body. The action of breathing, and the process of gas exchange in the lungs, are commonly described as "respiration", and the organs, tissues, and structures that enable us to breathe as the "respiratory system".

What you will find in this chapter

This chapter gives first aid treatment for conditions that commonly affect the process of respiration. These include the various ways in which breathing may be impaired, such as airway obstruction (including choking); situations that prevent the normal exchange of gases taking place (for example, inhalation of fumes); and emergencies caused by conditions that affect the lungs, and hence the physical process of breathing (for example, drowning and asthma).

CONTENTS

THE FIRST AIDER SHOULD:

• Recognise respiratory distress.

• Restore and maintain the casualty's breathing, using, if necessary, the ABC of resuscitation.

• Remove the cause of the problem and provide fresh air.

• Obtain appropriate medical aid. Any casualty who has experienced severe airway or breathing difficulties *must* be seen at hospital, even if first aid treatment appears to have been successful.

THE RESPIRATORY SYSTEM

We breathe air in and out in order to take oxygen into the lungs, and to expel the waste gas carbon dioxide, a by-product of *respiration*. Breathing is not quite the same as respiration, which is the process whereby oxygen and carbon dioxide are exchanged in the lungs, and in the cells of the body. (The process of gas exchange within the body tissues is described in *The Circulatory System*, on page 66.)

When we breathe in, air is drawn in at the nose and mouth, and passes down the main airway to the lungs. Within the lungs, it travels along a broadening network of air passages that finally open into tiny air sacs (*alveoli*). Here, the oxygen is taken up by the blood. Carbon dioxide-bearing air is then expelled as we breathe out, enabling fresh oxygen-bearing air to be drawn in with the next breath.

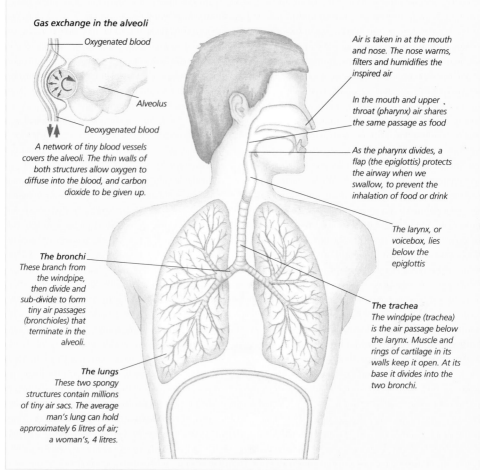

Gas exchange in the alveoli

Oxygenated blood

Alveolus

Deoxygenated blood

A network of tiny blood vessels covers the alveoli. The thin walls of both structures allow oxygen to diffuse into the blood, and carbon dioxide to be given up.

The bronchi
These branch from the windpipe, then divide and sub-divide to form tiny air passages (bronchioles) that terminate in the alveoli.

The lungs
These two spongy structures contain millions of tiny air sacs. The average man's lung can hold approximately 6 litres of air; a woman's, 4 litres.

Air is taken in at the mouth and nose. The nose warms, filters and humidifies the inspired air

In the mouth and upper throat (pharynx) air shares the same passage as food

As the pharynx divides, a flap (the epiglottis) protects the airway when we swallow, to prevent the inhalation of food or drink

The larynx, or voicebox, lies below the epiglottis

The trachea
The windpipe (trachea) is the air passage below the larynx. Muscle and rings of cartilage in its walls keep it open. At its base it divides into the two bronchi.

HOW WE BREATHE

Breathing consists of three phases: breathing in (*inspiration*), breathing out (*expiration*), and a pause.

When we breathe in, muscles in the chest work to expand its volume, drawing air into the lungs. When we breathe out, the elastic chest wall regains its resting position, and the air is pushed out. Some air is always left in the lungs so that oxygen is constantly available to the blood.

What controls breathing?

Breathing is controlled by the respiratory centre in the brain. No conscious effort is required to breathe, though in normal circumstances we can change the depth and rate of breathing voluntarily. An adult normally breathes about 16 times per minute; children breathe 20–30 times per minute. The rate may be altered (usually increased) by the respiratory centre as a response to stress, exercise, injury, or illness.

The composition of air

Air is a mixture of gases, of which 80 per cent is nitrogen and 20 per cent is oxygen. Only some of this oxygen is used up by respiration, so the air we breathe out still contains 16 per cent oxygen, in addition to a small amount of carbon dioxide. The oxygen level in exhaled air is thus adequate to resuscitate another person.

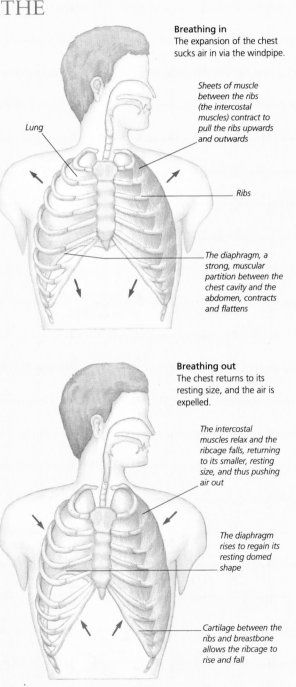

Breathing in
The expansion of the chest sucks air in via the windpipe.

Sheets of muscle between the ribs (the intercostal muscles) contract to pull the ribs upwards and outwards

Lung

Ribs

The diaphragm, a strong, muscular partition between the chest cavity and the abdomen, contracts and flattens

Breathing out
The chest returns to its resting size, and the air is expelled.

The intercostal muscles relax and the ribcage falls, returning to its smaller, resting size, and thus pushing air out

The diaphragm rises to regain its resting domed shape

Cartilage between the ribs and breastbone allows the ribcage to rise and fall

DISORDERS OF RESPIRATION

Any disturbance of the respiratory process is potentially fatal, since it may lead to *asphyxia*. This is the medical term for suffocation, caused not only by smothering, but by any condition that prevents oxygen being taken up by the blood.

The depletion of oxygen in the body is known as *hypoxia*. In this state the tissues deteriorate very rapidly – brain cells start to die if their oxygen supply is interrupted for as little as three minutes.

Symptoms and signs of low blood oxygen

- Rapid, distressed breathing and gasping.
- Confusion, irritability, and aggression, leading to unconsciousness.
- Usually, blueness of the skin (*cyanosis*).
- If hypoxia is not swiftly reversed, breathing and the heart may stop.

Giving oxygen

Light, portable oxygen equipment is now widely available, and many First Aiders receive training in its use. It can be used to supplement artificial ventilation, or to enrich inhaled air for casualties who can breathe ("oxygen therapy"). If properly administered by a trained person, oxygen can do no harm.

Using oxygen apparatus safely

Always observe the following rules:
- Do not smoke or allow any naked flames in the vicinity of oxygen.
- Do not use any oils or greases on the control knobs or valves.
- Keep equipment in good order.
- Make sure the apparatus is checked over and recharged after use.

CONDITIONS CAUSING HYPOXIA (LOW BLOOD OXYGEN)

Condition	Causes
Insufficient oxygen in inspired air	Suffocation by smoke or gas • Changes in atmospheric pressure, as at high altitude, or in a depressurised aircraft
Airway obstruction	Suffocation by an external obstruction, such as a pillow, or water (drowning) • Blockage or swelling in the air passages • Compression of the windpipe; for example, caused by hanging or strangulation
Conditions affecting the chest wall	Crushing, for example by a fall of earth or sand, or pressure from a crowd • Chest wall injury with multiple rib fractures or constricting burns
Impaired lung function	Lung injury • Collapsed lung • Lung infections, such as pneumonia
Damage to the brain or nerves that control respiration	A head injury, or stroke, that damages the breathing centre in the brain • Some forms of poisoning • Paralysis of nerves controlling the muscles of breathing, as in spinal cord injury
Impaired oxygen uptake by the tissues	Carbon monoxide poisoning • Cyanide poisoning

AIRWAY OBSTRUCTION

The airway may be obstructed by food, vomit, or other foreign material, by swelling of the throat after injury, or, in an unconscious casualty, by the tongue. A child may inhale a foreign body that can block the lower air passages, or swell within the lung, possibly resulting in a collapsed lung (*see page 62*) or pneumonia.

General signs of an obstructed airway

• Noisy, laboured breathing.
• Reversed movement of the chest and abdomen: the chest wall will suck in and the abdomen will push out.
• Blueness of the skin (*cyanosis*).
• Flaring of the nostrils.
• Drawing in of the chest wall between the ribs and the soft spaces above the collar bone and breastbone.

See also: Burns to the mouth and throat, *page 107.*
Inhaled foreign body, *page 178.*
Opening the airway, *page 28.*
Unconsciousness, *page 115.*

SUFFOCATION

This occurs when air is prevented from reaching the lungs, either because there is a physical barrier that prevents air entering the nose or mouth, or because the air the casualty breathes is full of fumes or smoke.

See also: Inhalation of fumes, *page 61.*

TREATMENT

> YOUR AIMS ARE:
> • To restore a supply of fresh air to the casualty's lungs.
> • To seek medical aid.

1 Remove any obstruction to breathing, or move the casualty into fresh air.

Clear heavy debris from the chest to allow it to rise normally

IF she is unconscious, check breathing and pulse, and be prepared to resuscitate. Dial 999 for an ambulance, and place her in the recovery position (*see page 30*).

2 If she is conscious, reassure her, but keep her under observation. Call a doctor or an ambulance.

Quickly free the mouth and nose, and clear the mouth of any obstruction

CHOKING

A foreign object sticking at the back of the throat may either block the throat, or induce muscular spasm. This is known as choking. Adults may choke on a piece of food that has been inadequately chewed and hurriedly swallowed. Young children like putting objects inside their mouths; boiled sweets are a particular danger.

RECOGNITION

There will be:
- Difficulty in speaking and breathing.

There may be:
- Blueness of the skin (*cyanosis*).
- Signs from the casualty – pointing to the throat, or grasping the neck.

TREATMENT

YOUR AIM IS:
- To remove the obstruction and restore normal breathing.

FOR AN ADULT

1 Dial 999 for an ambulance.

2 Give 6–10 abdominal thrusts. The obstruction may be expelled by the sudden pull against the diaphragm. Then check if the airway is clear.

3 Continue with sets of 6–10 abdominal thrusts.

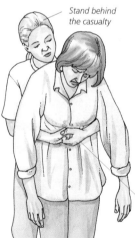

Stand behind the casualty

Interlock your hands and pull sharply inwards and upwards

4 If the casualty becomes unconscious, lay her face up on the floor. Kneel astride her and perform abdominal thrusts.

IF breathing returns, place her in the recovery position. If it does not, begin resuscitation.

FOR A CASUALTY WHO BECOMES UNCONSCIOUS

1 Dial 999 for an ambulance.

2 Loss of consciousness may relieve muscle spasm, so check first to see if the casualty can now breathe. If not, attempt 2 rescue breaths.

3 If this fails, kneel astride the casualty, and perform 6–10 abdominal thrusts.

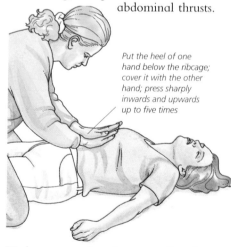

Put the heel of one hand below the ribcage; cover it with the other hand; press sharply inwards and upwards up to five times

IF she starts to breathe normally, place her in the recovery position (*see page 30*), and wait for the ambulance. Check and record breathing and pulse rate every 10 minutes.

IF she does not start to breathe again, begin resuscitation (*see page 38*).

FOR A CHILD

FOR A BABY

> DO NOT use your fingers to feel blindly down the throat.

Children under school age
Perform first aid for choking on children of 1–3 years of age just as you would for adults and older children – except do not perform blind finger sweeps. Instead, use your finger to sweep out the foreign body only if you can see it.

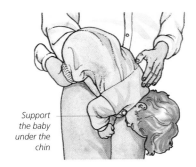

Support the baby under the chin

1 Dial 999 for an ambulance.

2 Give 6–10 abdominal thrusts. The obstruction may be expelled by the sudden pull against the diaphragm. Then check if the airway is clear.

3 Continue with sets of 6–10 abdominal thrusts.

4 If the casualty becomes unconscious, lay him face up on the floor and give 2 rescue breaths. If unsuccessful, kneel astride him and perform abdominal thrusts.

IF breathing returns, place him in the recovery position and wait for the ambulance. If it does not, begin resuscitation (*see pages 36–38*).

1 Lay the baby face down along your forearm and give five sharp slaps on the back (*see above*).

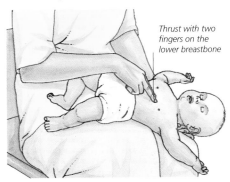

Thrust with two fingers on the lower breastbone

2 If this fails, turn her face up your other arm, or your lap, and give five sharp thrusts to the lower breastbone, using two fingers only (*see below*).

3 Check the mouth and remove any object you can *see*. Repeat the whole process as often as necessary.

IF the baby becomes unconscious, begin resuscitation and call an ambulance.

> DO NOT use abdominal thrusts on a baby.

DROWNING

Death by drowning usually occurs not because the lungs are full of water, but because throat spasm prevents breathing. Usually only a relatively small amount of water enters the lungs. The water that often gushes out of a rescued casualty's mouth comes from the stomach, rather than the lungs, and should be allowed to drain naturally. Attempts to force water from the stomach may result in stomach contents being inhaled. A drowned casualty may be suffering the effects of cold as well as asphyxia and may need to be treated for hypothermia.

The casualty should always receive medical attention. Any water entering the lungs will cause irritation and, even if the casualty appears to recover rapidly and fully at the time, swelling of the air passages ("secondary drowning") may still develop some hours later.

See also: Hypothermia, *page 130.*
Rescue from drowning, *page 24.*

TREATMENT

> YOUR AIMS ARE:
> • To prevent and treat low blood oxygen.
> • To arrange removal to hospital.

> DO NOT use the abdominal thrust unless the airway is blocked.

1 If carrying the casualty, keep his head lower than the rest of the body to reduce the risk of inhaling water.

2 Lay him down on a coat or blanket. Open the airway, check breathing and pulse, and be prepared to resuscitate if necessary.

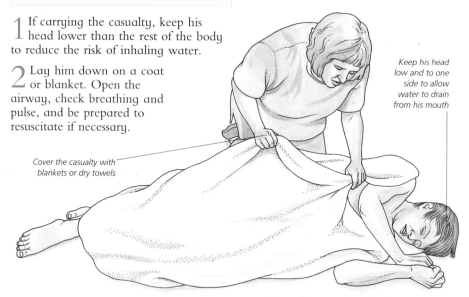

Keep his head low and to one side to allow water to drain from his mouth

Cover the casualty with blankets or dry towels

• Water in the lungs and the effects of cold can increase resistance to artificial ventilation and chest compression, so you may have to perform both at a slower rate than normal.

3 Treat the casualty for hypothermia: replace wet clothing, insulate him from the cold, and give him hot drinks.

4 Take or send the casualty to hospital, even if he appears to recover fully.

HANGING, STRANGLING, AND THROTTLING

Pressure on the outside of the neck squeezes the airway and blocks the flow of air to the lungs.
- *Hanging* is suspension of the body by a noose around the neck.
- *Strangling* occurs when the air supply is cut off by a constriction around the neck.
- *Throttling* is cutting off the air supply by squeezing a person's throat.

Hanging and strangulation may occur accidentally – for example, by a tie or clothing caught in machinery. Hanging may also cause a broken neck.

RECOGNITION

There may be:
- A constricting article around the neck.
- Marks around the casualty's neck where a constriction has been removed.
- Rapid, distressed breathing, impaired consciousness, and blueness of the skin (*cyanosis*).
- Congestion of the face, with prominent veins and, possibly, tiny red spots on the face or on the whites of the eyes.

See also: Spinal injury, *page 154.*

TREATMENT

YOUR AIMS ARE:
- To restore adequate breathing.
- To arrange removal to hospital.

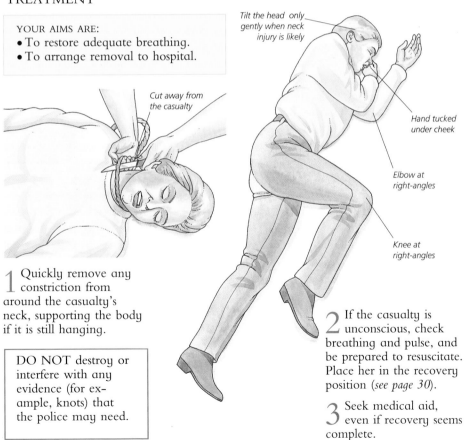

Tilt the head only gently when neck injury is likely

Cut away from the casualty

Hand tucked under cheek

Elbow at right-angles

Knee at right-angles

1 Quickly remove any constriction from around the casualty's neck, supporting the body if it is still hanging.

DO NOT destroy or interfere with any evidence (for example, knots) that the police may need.

2 If the casualty is unconscious, check breathing and pulse, and be prepared to resuscitate. Place her in the recovery position (*see page 30*).

3 Seek medical aid, even if recovery seems complete.

59

INHALATION OF FUMES

The inhalation of smoke, gases, or toxic vapours can be lethal, and rescue attempts must not be made if they put your own life at risk. Smoke or fumes that have accumulated in a confined space may quickly overcome a rescuer who is not wearing protective equipment. A burning building presents additional hazards – not only the fire itself, but also, possibly, falling masonry or timber.

Smoke inhalation

Any person who has been enclosed in a confined space during a fire may have inhaled smoke. Smoke from burning plastics, foam padding, and synthetic wall coverings will contain poisonous fumes. Casualties should be examined for other injuries sustained as a result of the fire.

Carbon monoxide

This highly dangerous gas prevents the blood from carrying oxygen. A large amount in the air can very quickly prove fatal. However, lengthy exposure to a small amount of the gas – for example, a slow leak from a faulty gas heater – may also cause severe, possibly fatal poisoning.

See also: Fires, *page 20.*
Burns to the mouth and throat, *page 107.*
Unconsciousness, *page 115.*

THE EFFECTS OF FUME INHALATION

Gas	Source	Effects
Smoke	Fires: smoke is low in oxygen, which is used up in combustion, and may contain other toxic fumes from burning materials	Irritation of the air passages causing spasm and swelling, resulting in rapid, noisy, distressed breathing, with coughing and wheezing • Unconsciousness • Burning in or around the nose or mouth
Carbon monoxide	Exhaust fumes of motor vehicles; the smoke from most fires; back-draughts from blocked chimney flues; and emissions from defective gas or paraffin heaters	• Chronic exposure may produce headache, confusion, aggression, nausea, vomiting, and incontinence • Acute poisoning may produce rapid, distressed breathing, blueness of the skin (*cyanosis*), and impaired consciousness leading rapidly to unconsciousness
Carbon dioxide	Tends to accumulate and become dangerously concentrated in deep enclosed spaces, such as pits, wells, and underground tanks	Breathlessness • Headache • Dizziness, leading rapidly to unconsciousness
Solvents	Glues and cleaning fluids. Abusers often use a plastic bag to concentrate the vapour	Headache • Vomiting • Stupor, leading to unconsciousness • Death may be caused by cardiac arrest, by choking on vomit or, in an abuser, asphyxiation by a plastic bag
Fuels	Lighter fuels, camping gas, and propane-fuelled stoves	When discharged from their containers these gases are extremely cold and, if inhaled, can cause cardiac arrest

TREATMENT FOR SMOKE INHALATION

YOUR AIMS ARE:
- To restore adequate breathing.
- To obtain urgent medical attention.

1 Dial 999, asking for both fire and ambulance services.

2 Remove the casualty from danger and into fresh air. Extinguish any fire or smouldering on clothing (*see page 21*).

DO NOT enter a smoke-filled room without proper safety equipment.

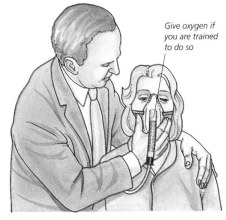

Give oxygen if you are trained to do so

IF she is unconscious, check breathing and pulse, and be prepared to resuscitate. Place her in the recovery position (*see page 30*).

3 Give oxygen if available, and if you have been trained in its use. Treat any burns (*see page 106*) or other injuries.

TREATMENT FOR FUME AND GAS INHALATION

YOUR AIMS ARE:
- To restore adequate breathing.
- To obtain urgent medical attention.

1 Dial 999, asking for both fire and ambulance services.

IF the casualty is unconscious, check breathing and pulse, and be prepared to resuscitate if necessary. Place her in the recovery position (*see page 30*).

3 Give oxygen if available, and if you have been trained in its use.

4 Stay with the casualty. Check and record breathing, pulse, and level of response every 10 minutes (*see page 50*).

Drag the casualty to safety

DO NOT enter a gas-filled room without a quick and easy means of escape.

2 If you are sure that it is safe to do so, remove the casualty from danger and into fresh air.

BREATHING DIFFICULTIES

These may be caused by chronic illness (conditions such as emphysema), by infections in the respiratory system (for example, croup or bronchitis), and by allergic reactions, either respiratory (for example, hay fever), or general-ised (*anaphylactic shock*).

Sudden attacks may be the result of psychological stress (*hyperventilation*), chest injury (*see right*), or the condition *asthma*. Prompt first aid can do much to help breathing and ease distress.

See also: Anaphylactic shock, *page 71.*

Collapsed lung *(pneumothorax)*

If air enters the space occupied by a lung, it will interfere with breathing, and may cause the lung to collapse. This can occur as a result of a wound that penetrates the chest wall (*see page 88*), or can happen spontaneously, because of a weakness of the lung itself. The pressure of air may also affect the action of the sound lung and the heart.

If you suspect a collapsed lung, help the casualty into the position in which he or she can breathe most easily, and call an ambulance without delay.

HYPERVENTILATION

The condition of over-breathing (hyper-ventilation) is commonly a manifestation of acute anxiety and may accompany hysteria or a panic attack. It is sometimes seen in susceptible individuals who have had a fright or a shock.

The excessive breathing causes chem-ical changes in the blood that produce the symptoms and signs of the condition. As breathing returns to normal, the casualty will gradually recover.

RECOGNITION

There will be:
• Unnaturally fast, deep breathing.

There may be:
• Attention-seeking behaviour.
• Dizziness, faintness, trembling, or marked tingling in the hands.
• Cramps in the hands and feet.

See also: Hysteria, *page 186.*

TREATMENT

YOUR AIM IS:
• To remove the casualty from any cause of distress, and calm her down.

1 Speak to the casualty firmly, but kindly.

2 If possible, lead her away to a quiet place, where she may be better able to regain control of her breathing.

3 Advise her to see her own doctor, to treat any underlying state of anxiety.

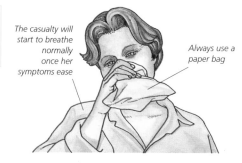

The casualty will start to breathe normally once her symptoms ease

Always use a paper bag

IF tingling or cramps persist, let her re-breathe her expired air from a paper bag.

ASTHMA

This is a distressing condition in which the muscles of the air passages go into spasm and constrict, making breathing (particularly breathing out) very difficult. Asthma attacks can be triggered by an allergy, or nervous tension. Often there is no obvious cause. Many sufferers are prone to sudden attacks at night.

Regular asthma sufferers generally know how best to cope with an attack. They usually carry medication in the form of a "puffer" aerosol. The majority of these drugs act to dilate the air passages, easing breathing.

RECOGNITION

There will be:
• Difficulty in breathing, with a markedly prolonged breathing-out phase.

There may be:
• Wheezing as the casualty breathes out.
• Distress and anxiety; the casualty may speak only with difficulty and in whispers.
• Blueness of the skin (*cyanosis*).
• In a severe attack, the effort of breathing will exhaust the casualty. Rarely, he or she may become unconscious, and stop breathing altogether.

TREATMENT

> YOUR AIM IS:
> • To ease breathing.
> • To seek medical aid if necessary.

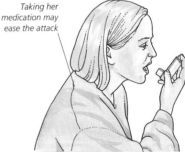
Taking her medication may ease the attack

1 Reassure and calm the casualty.

2 Help her to sit down, leaning slightly forward and resting on a support. Ensure a good supply of fresh air.

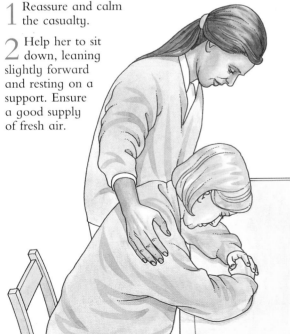

3 If the casualty has medication, let her use it.

IF the attack is a first attack, is prolonged, or does not respond to medication, or if the casualty is in severe respiratory distress, dial 999 for an ambulance. Check and record the casualty's breathing and pulse rate every 10 minutes.

IF the attack is mild and eases, the casualty should not need immediate medical attention, but should be encouraged to tell her doctor of the attack.

CROUP

This term describes attacks of severe breathing difficulty in very young children, caused by inflammation in the windpipe and larynx. Croup can be alarming, but almost always passes without causing lasting harm. It usually occurs at night and may recur before the child settles.

If the attack persists or is very severe, and is accompanied by fever, call an ambulance. There is a small risk that the child is suffering a rare croup-like condition, *epiglottitis*. In this condition, a small flap-like structure in the throat, the epiglottis (*see page 52*), becomes infected and swollen, sometimes so much so that it blocks the airway completely. The child thus needs urgent medical attention.

RECOGNITION

There will be:
• Distressed breathing in a young child.

There may be:
• A short, barking cough.
• A crowing or whistling noise, especially on breathing in (*stridor*).
• A blue colour to the skin (*cyanosis*).
• In severe cases, the child will be using muscles around the nose, neck, and upper arms, trying to breathe.

Suspect epiglottitis if:
• An older child is sitting bolt upright, evidently in severe respiratory distress.
• The child has a high temperature.

TREATMENT

YOUR AIMS ARE:
• To comfort and support the child.
• To seek medical advice.

DO NOT stick your fingers down the child's throat. This can produce spasm that may block the airway.

DO NOT panic. It will alarm the child, and worsen the attack.

1 Sit the child up, supporting her back, and reassure her.

2 Make the child breathe in steam to ease her breathing.
• Take her into the bathroom or kitchen and run the hot tap, or boil water.
• Try to create a humid atmosphere in the room where the child is put back to rest. This may prevent the attack recurring.

3 Call your doctor or, if croup is severe, dial 999 for an ambulance.

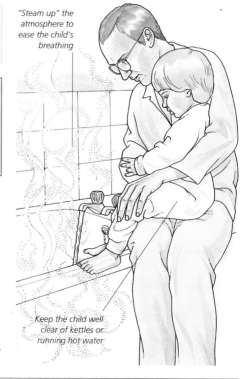

"Steam up" the atmosphere to ease the child's breathing

Keep the child well clear of kettles or running hot water

DISORDERS OF THE CIRCULATION

The heart and network of blood vessels, together known as the circulatory (or *cardiovascular*) system, work continuously to keep all parts of the body supplied with the vital oxygen and nutrients carried in the blood.

The system can fail for two main reasons. First, severe bleeding may cause the volume of circulating blood to fall, and deprive the vital organs – the brain, heart, and lungs – of oxygen. Secondly, age or disease can cause the system to break down.

What you will find in this chapter

The first aid techniques described in this chapter concentrate on improving the blood supply to the heart and brain. In minor incidents, such as a faint, this should ensure recovery; in serious cases such as heart attack, the First Aider's role may be essential in preserving life until medical aid is obtained.

THE FIRST AIDER SHOULD:

• Position the casualty to improve the blood supply to the vital organs. With heart disorders, this must be balanced against the risk of putting extra strain on the heart.

• Take any additional measures to improve the circulation and breathing – for example, loosening tight clothing.

• Comfort and reassure the casualty. Fear and panic will put extra strain on the heart.

• Obtain appropriate medical assistance. Always advise a casualty to inform his or her doctor of, for example, an angina attack or unexplained faint; never hesitate to call an ambulance if you suspect a more serious emergency.

CONTENTS

THE CIRCULATORY SYSTEM

Blood circulates around the body in a continuous cycle, pumped by the rhythmic contraction/relaxation, or beat, of the heart muscle. The blood circulates within a network of flexible tubes, known as blood vessels. There are three types of blood vessel: arteries, veins, and capillaries. The force with which the heart pumps the blood through the vessels and around the body is known as the "blood pressure". The circulating blood distributes oxygen and nutrients to the tissues, and carries waste products away.

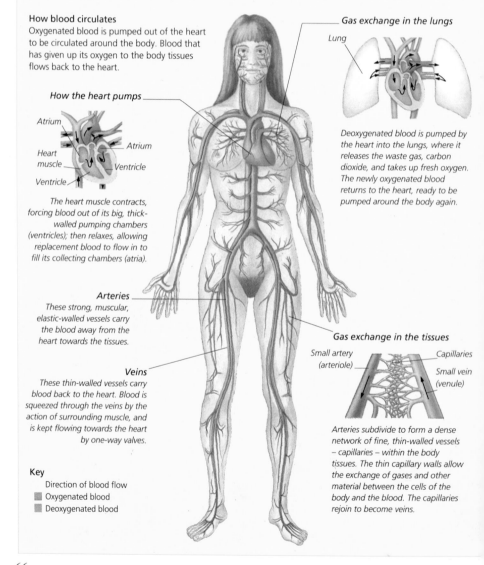

How blood circulates
Oxygenated blood is pumped out of the heart to be circulated around the body. Blood that has given up its oxygen to the body tissues flows back to the heart.

How the heart pumps

Atrium

Atrium

Heart muscle

Ventricle

Ventricle

The heart muscle contracts, forcing blood out of its big, thick-walled pumping chambers (ventricles); then relaxes, allowing replacement blood to flow in to fill its collecting chambers (atria).

Arteries
These strong, muscular, elastic-walled vessels carry the blood away from the heart towards the tissues.

Veins
These thin-walled vessels carry blood back to the heart. Blood is squeezed through the veins by the action of surrounding muscle, and is kept flowing towards the heart by one-way valves.

Key
Direction of blood flow
Oxygenated blood
Deoxygenated blood

Gas exchange in the lungs

Lung

Deoxygenated blood is pumped by the heart into the lungs, where it releases the waste gas, carbon dioxide, and takes up fresh oxygen. The newly oxygenated blood returns to the heart, ready to be pumped around the body again.

Gas exchange in the tissues

Small artery (arteriole)

Capillaries

Small vein (venule)

Arteries subdivide to form a dense network of fine, thin-walled vessels – capillaries – within the body tissues. The thin capillary walls allow the exchange of gases and other material between the cells of the body and the blood. The capillaries rejoin to become veins.

Composition of the blood

There are about six litres (10 pints) of blood in the average adult body. It consists of a clear yellow fluid (*plasma*) in which are suspended red blood cells, white blood cells, and platelets. Blood is made up of approximately two-thirds plasma and one-third cells.

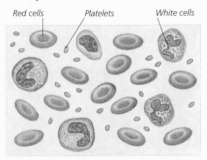

Red cells   Platelets   White cells

The blood cells
Red blood cells contain haemoglobin, a red pigment that combines readily with oxygen. The white cells help the body to fight infection. Platelets help the blood to clot (*see page 77*).

What can go wrong

• The amount of oxygen carried in the blood may be reduced, by a deficiency in the red blood cells (*anaemia*), or by an insufficiency of oxygen available in the lungs (*see page 54*). Anaemia makes the skin pale (*pallor*); blood low in oxygen gives a blue tinge to the skin (*cyanosis*).

• Continuously high blood pressure, produced by conditions such as hardening of the arteries (*arteriosclerosis*), may cause a blood vessel to rupture, resulting in internal bleeding.

• Poor circulation, hardened arteries, or narrowed blood vessels can contribute to the forming of a blood clot (*thrombosis*). The clot may travel within the circulatory system to lodge elsewhere. This is known as *embolism*.

• A fall in blood pressure (for example, due to bleeding) may prevent an adequate supply of blood, and therefore oxygen, to the vital organs. Shock (*see overleaf*) may develop.

THE PULSE

This is the wave of pressure that passes along the arteries, created by each beat of the heart. It can normally be felt where an artery passes close to the surface of the body. In adults, the pulse rate is usually between 60 and 80 beats per minute. It is faster in children, and may be slower in very fit adults. The pulse rate may increase with exertion, fear, fever, blood loss and some illnesses. Fainting, certain heart disorders, and cerebral compression may slow it down.

Where the pulse may be felt

The pulse is most commonly recorded at the wrist (the *radial* pulse). In an emergency the neck, or *carotid*, pulse is used (*see page 29*). In babies, the *brachial* pulse (*see page 36*), on the inside of the upper arm, may be easier to find.

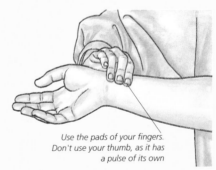

Use the pads of your fingers. Don't use your thumb, as it has a pulse of its own

To take the radial pulse, place three fingers in the hollow immediately above the wrist creases at the base of the thumb, and press lightly.
Check and record:

• Rate (beats per minute);

• Strength (strong or weak);

• Rhythm (regular or irregular).

SHOCK

The function of the circulatory system is to distribute blood to all parts of the body, so that the oxygen and nutrients it carries can pass through, or "perfuse", the tissues. When the system fails, and insufficient oxygen reaches the tissues, the medical condition known as shock will develop.

If shock is not swiftly treated, the vital organs can fail, leading ultimately to death. You should note that the condition is made worse by fear and pain.

What causes shock?

First, shock can develop when the heart pump fails to do its work, so that the pressure of the circulating blood is reduced. The most common cause of this type of shock is a heart attack.

Secondly, shock may develop when the volume of fluid circulating around the body is reduced. External or internal bleeding, or loss of other bodily fluids through severe diarrhoea, vomiting, or burns, are the most common examples. The body responds by withdrawing the blood supply from the surface to the core of the body. The main symptoms and signs of shock relate to this redistribution of the circulation.

RECOGNITION

At first, a flow of adrenaline causes:
• A rapid pulse.
• Pale, grey skin, especially inside the lips. A fingernail or earlobe, if pressed, will not regain its colour immediately.
• Sweating, and cold, clammy skin, because the sweat does not evaporate.

As shock develops, there may be:
• Weakness and giddiness.
• Nausea, and possibly vomiting.
• Thirst.
• Rapid, shallow breathing.
• A weak "thready" pulse. When the pulse at the wrist disappears, fluid loss may equal half the blood volume.

As the oxygen supply to the brain weakens:
• The casualty may become restless, anxious and even aggressive.
• The casualty may yawn and gasp for air (this is known as "air hunger").
• The casualty will become unconscious.
• Finally, the heart will stop.

See also: Severe external
   bleeding, *page 78.*
   Severe burns, *page 106.*
   Unconsciousness, *page 116.*

HOW THE BODY RESPONDS TO BLOOD LOSS

Approximate volume	Effect on the body
½ litre (1 pint)	Little or no effect; this is the quantity normally taken in a blood donor session.
2 litres (3½ pints)	The hormone adrenaline is released, quickening the pulse, and inducing sweating. Small blood vessels in non-vital areas, such as the skin, are shut down to divert blood, and the oxygen it carries, to the vital organs. Shock will become evident.
3 litres (5 pints)	As blood loss approaches this level (half the normal volume), the pulse at the wrist may become undetectable.The casualty will usually lose consciousness; breathing and the heart may stop.

TREATMENT

YOUR AIMS ARE:
• To recognise shock.
• To treat any obvious cause.
• To improve the blood supply to the brain, heart, and lungs.
• To arrange urgent removal to hospital.

DO NOT let the casualty move unnecessarily, eat, drink, or smoke. If he complains of thirst, moisten his lips with water.

DO NOT leave the casualty unattended. Reassure him constantly.

1 Treat any cause of shock you can remedy (such as external bleeding).

2 Lay the casualty down, keeping his head low.

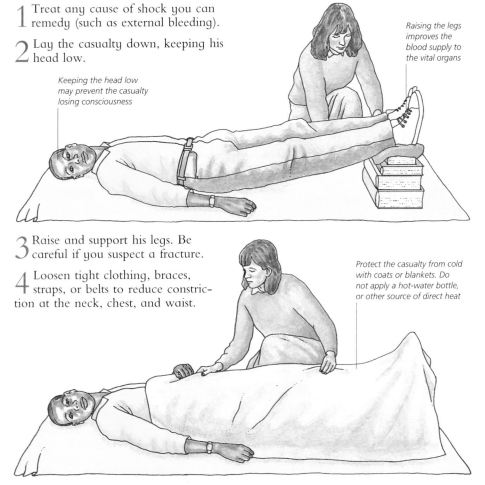

Raising the legs improves the blood supply to the vital organs

Keeping the head low may prevent the casualty losing consciousness

3 Raise and support his legs. Be careful if you suspect a fracture.

4 Loosen tight clothing, braces, straps, or belts to reduce constriction at the neck, chest, and waist.

Protect the casualty from cold with coats or blankets. Do not apply a hot-water bottle, or other source of direct heat

5 Insulate the casualty from cold, both above and below. Dial 999 for an ambulance.

6 Check and record breathing, pulse and level of response (*see page 50*). Be prepared to resuscitate if necessary.

FAINTING

A faint (also known as *syncope*) is a brief loss of consciousness caused by a temporary reduction of blood flow to the brain. Unlike shock, the pulse becomes very slow, though it soon picks up and returns to normal. Recovery is usually rapid and complete.

A faint may be a reaction to pain or fright, or the result of emotional upset, exhaustion, or lack of food. It is more common, however, after long periods of physical inactivity, especially in warm atmospheres. Blood pools in the lower part of the body, reducing the amount available to the brain.

RECOGNITION

There will be:
- A brief loss of consciousness; the casualty will fall to the floor.
- A slow pulse.
- Pallor.

See also: Unconsciousness, *page 115.*

TREATMENT

YOUR AIMS ARE:
- To improve blood flow to the brain.
- To reassure the casualty as she recovers, and make her comfortable.

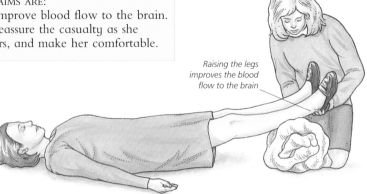

Raising the legs improves the blood flow to the brain

1 Lay the casualty down, and raise and support her legs.

2 Make sure she has plenty of fresh air; open a window if necessary.

3 As she recovers, reassure her and help her sit up gradually.

4 Look for and treat any injury sustained through falling.

IF she does not regain consciousness quickly, check breathing and pulse, and be prepared to resuscitate if necessary. Place her in the recovery position (*see page 30*) and dial 999 for an ambulance.

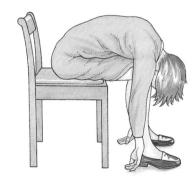

IF she starts to feel faint again, place her head between her knees and tell her to take deep breaths.

ANAPHYLACTIC SHOCK

This is the name given to a massive allergic reaction within the body. It is a serious, potentially fatal condition that may develop, in sensitive individuals, within a few seconds or minutes of:
• The injection of a particular drug.
• The sting of a particular insect.
• The ingestion of a particular food.
The reaction causes substances to be released into the blood that dilate blood vessels and constrict air passages. Blood pressure falls dramatically, and breathing becomes difficult. Swelling of the face and neck increases the risk of suffocation.
The amount of oxygen reaching the vital organs becomes severely reduced. The casualty urgently needs oxygen and a life-saving injection of adrenaline. There is no specific first aid treatment beyond assisting breathing and minimising shock until specialised help arrives.

RECOGNITION

There may be:
• Anxiety.
• Widespread red, blotchy skin eruption.
• Swelling of the face and neck.
• Puffiness around the eyes.
• Impaired breathing, ranging from a tight chest to severe difficulty; the casualty may wheeze and gasp for air.
• A rapid pulse.

See also: Allergy, *page 187.*

TREATMENT

YOUR AIM IS:
• To arrange urgent removal to hospital.

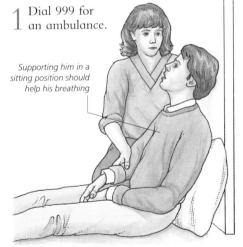

1 Dial 999 for an ambulance.

Supporting him in a sitting position should help his breathing

2 Help a conscious casualty sit up in the position which most relieves any breathing difficulty.

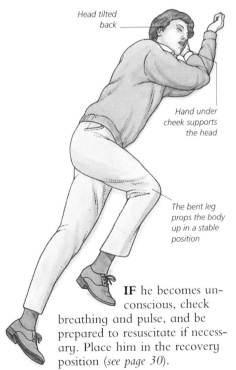

Head tilted back

Hand under cheek supports the head

The bent leg props the body up in a stable position

IF he becomes unconscious, check breathing and pulse, and be prepared to resuscitate if necessary. Place him in the recovery position (*see page 30*).

DISORDERS OF THE HEART

The heart is a very specialised pump whose muscle, the *myocardium*, "beats" throughout our lives in a continuous, smooth and co-ordinated way, controlled by an electrical impulse.

The heart muscle has its own blood supply, provided by the *coronary arteries* (so-called because they encircle the heart like a crown). Like all other arteries, these are susceptible to narrowing and blockage. In severe cases, or if the electrical impulse is disrupted, the heart may stop (*cardiac arrest*).

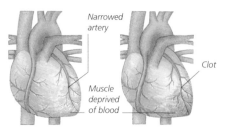
Narrowed artery

Clot

Muscle deprived of blood

Narrowed artery
Insufficient oxygen is delivered to an area of heart muscle. This is the cause of the condition *angina pectoris*.

Blocked artery
A clot may form in an artery, or travel from elsewhere. Part of the heart muscle is deprived of oxygen, and may die.

ANGINA PECTORIS

The name means a crushing of the chest, and describes the pain experienced when narrowed coronary arteries are unable to deliver sufficient blood to the heart muscle to meet the extra demands of exertion or, sometimes, of excitement. An attack will force the casualty to rest, whereupon the pain should soon ease.

RECOGNITION

There may be:
- Gripping chest pain, often spreading to the left arm and jaw.
- Pain or tingling in the hand.
- Shortness of breath.
- Weakness, often sudden and extreme.

TREATMENT

YOUR AIM IS:
- To ease strain on the heart by ensuring that the casualty rests.

1 Help the casualty sit down. Reassure him, and make him comfortable.

2 If the casualty has medicine for angina, help him to take it.

The casualty may have tablets or a "puffer" aerosol to ease an attack

Help the casualty to ensure that he rests

3 Let the casualty rest. The attack should settle within a few minutes, or in response to the drug.

IF pain persists or returns, dial 999 for an ambulance. Monitor breathing and pulse, and be prepared to resuscitate if necessary.

HEART ATTACK

A heart attack most commonly occurs when the blood supply to part of the heart muscle is suddenly obstructed – for example, by a clot in one of the coronary arteries (*coronary thrombosis*). The effect depends largely on how much of the heart muscle is affected. Many casualties recover completely.

Drugs that aid recovery include special medicines called *thrombolytics*, which dissolve the clot, and ordinary aspirin, which "thins" the blood. The main risk during any heart attack is that the heart will stop (*see* Cardiac Arrest, *overleaf*).

RECOGNITION

There may be:

- Persistent crushing, vice-like pain, often radiating from the heart. Unlike the pain of angina, it does not ease with rest, and indeed may occur at rest.
- Breathlessness, and discomfort high in the abdomen, like severe indigestion.
- Sudden faintness or giddiness.
- A sense of impending doom.
- "Ashen" skin, and blueness at the lips.
- A rapid pulse, becoming weaker.
- Collapse, often without any warning.

TREATMENT

YOUR AIMS ARE:
- To minimise the work of the heart.
- To summon urgent medical aid and arrange removal to hospital.

Help the casualty into a relaxed position to ease strain on the heart

1 Make the casualty comfortable. A half-sitting position, with head and shoulders supported and knees bent, is often best.

2 Dial 999 for an ambulance and say that you suspect a heart attack. If the casualty asks you to do so, call his own doctor also. Keep a constant check on pulse and breathing and be ready to resuscitate if necessary.

Give his knees and shoulders firm support

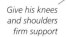

3 If you have ordinary aspirin and the casualty is conscious, give him one tablet and tell him to chew it slowly. This may help to limit the damage to the heart.

Acute heart failure

Heart failure is a condition in which the heart muscle is strained and fatigued – for example, following a coronary thrombosis. Acute attacks often occur at night. They may appear similar to an asthma attack (*see page 63*), with severe breathlessness, often, but not always, accompanied by other signs and symptoms of heart attack. Follow the treatment for heart attack.

CARDIAC ARREST

The term "cardiac arrest" describes any sudden stoppage of the heart. It may be the result of a heart attack; other causes include severe blood loss, suffocation, electric shock, anaphylactic shock, drug overdose, and hypothermia.

Cardiac arrest is characterised by the absence of pulse and breathing. You must commence resuscitation as soon as possible because, without oxygen, the heart muscle and brain will deteriorate rapidly. The ABC of resuscitation techniques is fully described in the chapter *Resuscitation (pages 25-38)*.

RECOGNITION

There will be:
- Absence of pulse.
- Absence of breathing.

TREATMENT

YOUR AIM IS:
- To keep the heart muscle and brain supplied with oxygen until an ambulance arrives.

1 Check for breathing and a pulse on any unconscious casualty.

2 If both are absent, dial 999 for an ambulance and begin the sequence of resuscitation (*see page 38*).

Ventricular fibrillation

This is the most common cause of sudden cardiac arrest. It is an electric storm that originates in a damaged ventricle, or one deprived of oxygen. The electrical heart impulse becomes chaotic, and the muscle fails to contract in harmony.

The use of defibrillators Ventricular fibrillation can often be reversed by the early application of a controlled electric shock from a machine called a defibrillator, now carried by most ambulances. The role of the First Aider is to keep the brain supplied with oxygen, by means of cardiopulmonary resuscitation, until a defibrillator can be brought to the casualty and used by a trained operator.

The defibrillator monitors the casualty's condition, and automatically indicates when a shock is advised

Electrodes attached to conductive pads must be correctly positioned on the casualty's chest

Everybody must be well clear of the casualty's body when a shock is delivered

WOUNDS AND BLEEDING

Any abnormal break in the skin or body surfaces is known as a wound. Most wounds are *open* – with a break in the skin through which blood and other fluids may be lost from the body, and germs may enter and cause infection. A *closed* wound allows blood to escape from the circulatory system, but not the body – the condition known as internal bleeding. The nature of the wounding force determines the type of wound and influences the treatment given.

What you will find in this chapter

This chapter covers first aid for all types of bleeding, from serious open wounds to minor bruises. Whatever the injury, you must maintain scrupulous hygiene, and also protect yourself from any infection that the casualty may be carrying in the bloodstream. More information on preventing cross-infection is given in the chapter *Dressings and Bandages (page 200)*. If you become concerned about disease transmission after having treated an open wound, consult your doctor.

THE FIRST AIDER SHOULD:

• Control blood loss by applying pressure over the wound and raising the injured part.

• Take steps to minimise shock, which may be caused by extensive blood loss.

• Protect the wound from infection, and promote natural healing, by covering it with a dressing.

• Since germs can be present in body fluids, at all times pay scrupulous attention to hygiene, both to protect the casualty and yourself.

CONTENTS

TYPES OF WOUND

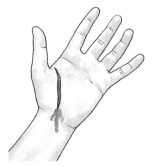

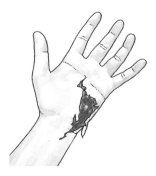

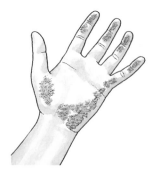

Incised wound
A clean cut from a sharp edge, such as a blade or broken glass. Because the blood vessels at the edges of the wound are cut straight across, there may be profuse bleeding. Incised wounds to a limb may also sever underlying structures such as tendons.

Laceration
A rough tear by crushing or ripping forces, such as machinery. Lacerations may bleed less profusely than clean-cut wounds, but there is more tissue damage and bruising. They are also often contaminated by germs; the risk of infection is high.

Abrasion (graze)
A superficial wound in which the top layers of skin are scraped off leaving a raw, tender area, most commonly caused by a sliding fall or a friction burn. Abrasions often contain embedded foreign particles that may cause infection.

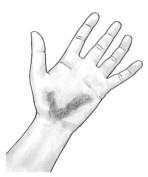

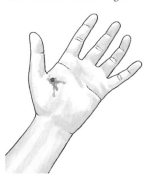

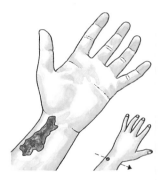

Contusion (bruise)
Any blunt blow (a punch, for example) can rupture capillaries beneath the skin. Blood leaks into the tissues, causing bruising. The skin may be split, but is often unbroken. Severe contusion may indicate deeper, hidden damage, such as a fracture or internal injury.

Puncture wound
Standing on a nail, being jabbed with a needle, or being stabbed, for example, result in puncture wounds, with a small site of entry but a deep track of internal damage. As dirt and germs can be carried far into the body, the risk of infection is very high.

Gunshot wound
A bullet or other missile may be driven into or through the body, causing serious internal injury and sucking in contaminants. The wound at the point of entry may be small and neat, but the exit wound, if there is one, may be large and ragged.

TYPES OF BLEEDING

Bleeding (*haemorrhage*) is classified according to the type of blood vessel that is damaged: artery, vein, or capillary (*see page 66*). Arterial bleeding can be very dramatic, but copious venous bleeding is potentially more serious.

Arterial bleeding

The blood, richly oxygenated, is bright red and, under pressure from the pumping heart, *spurts* from the wound in time with the heart beat. A severed artery may produce a jet of blood several feet high, and can rapidly empty the circulation of blood.

Venous bleeding

Venous blood, having given up its oxygen, is dark red in colour. It is under less pressure than arterial blood, but since the vein walls are capable of great distension, blood may "pool" within them; thus blood from a severed major vein may *gush* profusely.

Capillary bleeding

This type of bleeding, characterized as *oozing*, occurs at the site of all wounds. Although capillary bleeding may at first be brisk, blood loss is generally negligible. A blunt blow may rupture capillaries beneath the skin, causing bleeding into the tissues (a bruise).

How the body reacts to control bleeding

When blood vessels are severed or torn, their damaged ends constrict and retract in order to minimise blood loss. At the same time, the blood that escapes from damaged vessels begins to clot. Clotting is a complex process involving several factors, and if any one is absent (as in the condition *haemophilia*), clotting may be delayed.

If this local response is insufficient to contain blood loss, more general reactions causing changes in the circulatory system (*see page 68*) come into operation.

These diagrams show the principal stages in the formation of a blood clot.

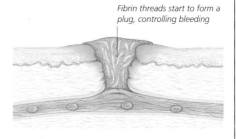

Fibrin threads start to form a plug, controlling bleeding

2 The fibrin forms a dense network that in turn traps more platelets, eventually forming a jelly-like clot. This normally takes about 10 minutes.

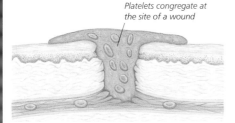

Platelets congregate at the site of a wound

1 Any damage to blood vessel walls causes platelets to congregate at the site of the injury. They not only help to plug the wound, but also release clotting factors that start to convert one of the blood substances, fibrinogen, into a protein, fibrin.

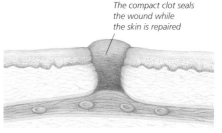

The compact clot seals the wound while the skin is repaired

3 The clot rapidly begins to shrink, releasing a watery substance (*serum*). This carries antibodies to combat infection, and specialised cells that begin the process of repair. Serum collects in the tissues around the injury, causing swelling.

SEVERE EXTERNAL BLEEDING

Massive external bleeding is dramatic and may distract you from first aid priorities; remember the ABC of resuscitation. Bleeding at the face or neck can obstruct the airway. Rarely, blood loss is so great that the heart stops. Remember, too, that shock may well develop and the casualty may lose consciousness.

See also: Shock, *page 68.*
Unconsciousness, *page 115.*

Protecting yourself

If you have any sores or open wounds, make sure that they are covered with a waterproof adhesive dressing. Use disposable gloves whenever possible, and wash your hands thoroughly in soap and water before, and after, treatment. More information on protecting yourself and the casualty from infection is given on page 200.

TREATMENT

YOUR AIMS ARE:
- To control the bleeding.
- To prevent shock.
- To minimise the risk of infection.
- To arrange urgent removal to hospital.

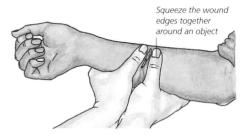

Squeeze the wound edges together around an object

1 Remove or cut clothing to expose the wound. Watch out for sharp objects, such as glass, that might injure you.

IF you cannot apply direct pressure – for example, if an object is protruding – press down firmly on either side.

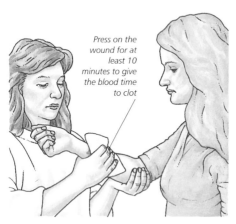

Press on the wound for at least 10 minutes to give the blood time to clot

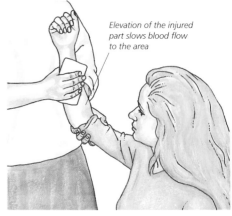

Elevation of the injured part slows blood flow to the area

2 Apply direct pressure over the wound with your fingers or palm, preferably over a sterile dressing or clean pad – but do not waste time hunting for a dressing.

3 Raise and support an injured limb above the level of the casualty's heart. Handle limbs very gently if the injury involves a fracture (*see page 141*).

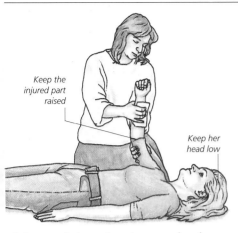

Keep the injured part raised

Keep her head low

4 It may help to lay the casualty down. This will reduce blood flow to the site of injury, and minimise shock.

5 Leaving any original pad in place, apply a sterile dressing. Bandage it in place firmly, but not so tightly as to impede the circulation (*see page 205*). If bleeding strikes through the dressing, bandage another firmly over the top.

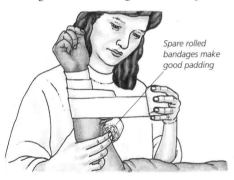

Spare rolled bandages make good padding

IF there is a protruding foreign body, build up pads on either side of the object until they are high enough to bandage over the object without pressing on it.

6 Secure and support the injured part as for a broken bone (*see page 141*).

7 Dial 999 for an ambulance. Treat the casualty for shock. Check the dressing for seepage, and check the circulation beyond the bandage.

Indirect pressure

Rarely, direct pressure is impossible to apply, or is insufficient to staunch bleeding from a limb. In these cases, indirect pressure may be applied to a "pressure point", where a main artery runs close to a bone. Pressure at these points will cut off the blood supply to the limb. It must not be applied for longer than 10 minutes.

DO NOT use a tourniquet. It can make the bleeding worse, and may result in tissue damage, and even gangrene.

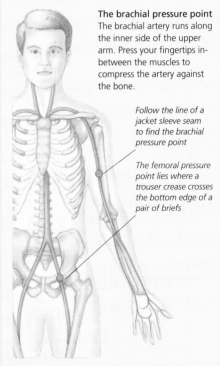

The brachial pressure point
The brachial artery runs along the inner side of the upper arm. Press your fingertips in-between the muscles to compress the artery against the bone.

Follow the line of a jacket sleeve seam to find the brachial pressure point

The femoral pressure point lies where a trouser crease crosses the bottom edge of a pair of briefs

The femoral pressure point
The femoral artery crosses the pelvic bone in the centre of the groin crease. Lay the casualty down with the knee bent to locate the groin fold, and press very firmly with your thumbs.

BLEEDING AT SPECIAL SITES

There are a number of wounds that require slight variations on the general rules of direct and indirect pressure if they are to be successfully treated. Blood loss from wounds at these special sites may be copious, and the casualty must be observed carefully for signs of shock.

SCALP WOUNDS

The scalp has a rich blood supply, and when it is damaged, the skin splits, producing a gaping wound. Bleeding may be profuse, and will often make the injury appear more alarming than it really is. However, a scalp wound may be part of a more serious underlying injury, such as a skull fracture; examine the casualty very carefully, particularly if he or she is elderly, or in cases where a serious head injury may be masked by alcohol or drug intoxication. If in doubt, follow the treatment for head injury.

See also: Head injuries, *page 117.*
   Shock, *page 68.*

TREATMENT

YOUR AIMS ARE:
- To control blood loss.
- To arrange transport to hospital.

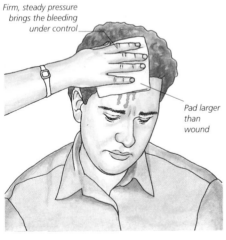

Firm, steady pressure brings the bleeding under control

Pad larger than wound

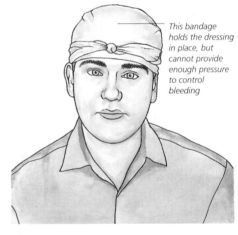

This bandage holds the dressing in place, but cannot provide enough pressure to control bleeding

1 Wearing disposable gloves, if possible, replace any displaced skin flaps.

2 Apply firm direct pressure over a sterile dressing or clean pad.

3 Secure the dressing using a triangular bandage (*see page 213*). If bleeding persists, reapply pressure on the pad.

4 Lay a conscious casualty down with his head and shoulders slightly raised; if he becomes unconscious, place him in the recovery position (*see page 30*).

5 Take or send the casualty to hospital in the treatment position.

WOUNDS TO THE PALM

The palm is richly supplied with blood, and a wound may bleed profusely. A deep wound may sever tendons and nerves, and result in loss of feeling in the fingers. If a foreign body prevents fist-clenching, use the treatment on page 95.

TREATMENT

YOUR AIMS ARE:
• To control blood loss.
• To arrange transport to hospital.

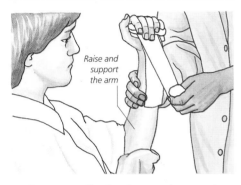

Raise and support the arm

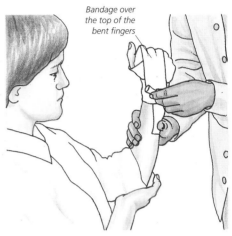

Bandage over the top of the bent fingers

1 Press a sterile dressing or clean pad firmly into the palm and ask the casualty to clench his fist over it. If he finds it difficult to press hard, he may grasp the fist with his uninjured hand.

2 Bandage the fingers so that they are clenched over the pad. Tie the knot over the fingers.

3 Support the arm in an elevation sling (see page 215), and take or send the casualty to hospital.

WOUNDS AT JOINT CREASES

Blood vessels crossing the inside of the elbow and knee pass near the surface and, if severed, will bleed copiously.

Remember that the technique below will, by compressing the artery, impede the blood supply to the lower part of the limb.

TREATMENT

YOUR AIMS ARE:
• To control blood loss.
• To arrange transport to hospital.

1 Press a clean pad over the injury. Bend the joint as firmly as possible.

2 Keeping the joint firmly bent to exert pressure over the pad, raise the limb. The casualty should lie down if necessary.

3 Take or send the casualty to hospital in the treatment position. Release the pressure briefly every 10 minutes to restore normal blood flow.

BLEEDING VARICOSE VEINS

Veins in the legs contain one-way valves that keep the blood flowing towards the heart. If these deteriorate, blood collects behind them, causing distension. The "varicose" vein has taut, thin walls and is often raised, stretching the skin (the characteristic "knobbly" appearance). It can be burst by surprisingly gentle knocks and will bleed profusely. If bleeding is not controlled, shock may develop.

See also: Shock, *page 68.*

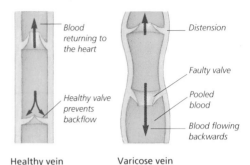

Blood returning to the heart

Healthy valve prevents backflow

Distension

Faulty valve

Pooled blood

Blood flowing backwards

Healthy vein   Varicose vein

TREATMENT

YOUR AIMS ARE:
- To bring blood loss under control.
- To arrange urgent removal to hospital.
- To minimise shock.

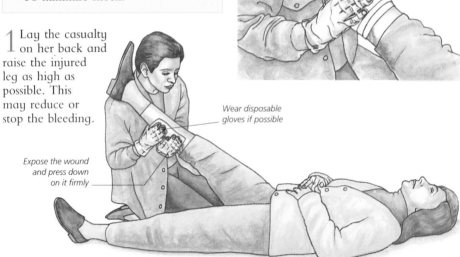

Keep the leg high

Wear disposable gloves if possible

1 Lay the casualty on her back and raise the injured leg as high as possible. This may reduce or stop the bleeding.

Expose the wound and press down on it firmly

2 Expose the site of the bleeding and apply firm direct pressure over a sterile dressing or clean pad, or with your fingers, until bleeding is controlled.

3 Remove garments such as garters or elastic-topped stockings that may be impeding blood flow back to the heart.

4 Place a large, soft pad over the dressing. Bandage it firmly to exert even pressure, but not so tightly that the circulation is impeded (*see page 205*).

5 Dial 999 for an ambulance. Keep the injured leg raised and supported until the ambulance arrives.

INTERNAL BLEEDING

Bleeding within the body cavities may follow injury, such as a fracture or penetrating wound, but can also occur spontaneously – for example, bleeding from a stomach ulcer. Internal bleeding is serious; although blood may not be spilt from the body, it is lost from the circulation, and shock can develop. In addition, accumulated blood can exert damaging pressure on organs such as the lungs or brain.

When to suspect internal bleeding

Suspect it if, following injury, signs of shock develop without obvious blood loss. At the site of violent injury, there may also be "pattern bruising" – discoloration that takes the pattern of clothes or crushing objects. There may be blood at body orifices (*see overleaf*), either fresh or mixed with the contents of injured organs.

RECOGNITION

There may be:
- Pallor.
- Cold, clammy skin.
- A rapid, weak pulse.
- Pain.
- Thirst.
- Confusion, restlessness, and irritability, possibly leading to collapse and unconsciousness.
- Information from the casualty indicating recent injury or illness, previous similar episodes, or drug-taking.
- After violent injury, pattern bruising.
- Bleeding from orifices (*see overleaf*).

See also: Cerebral compression, *page 119.*
Crush injuries, *page 92.*
Shock, *page 68.*
Unconsciousness, *page 115.*

TREATMENT

YOUR AIMS ARE:
- To arrange urgent removal to hospital.
- To minimise shock.

IF the casualty loses consciousness, place him in the recovery position (*see page 30*).

1 Help the casualty to lie down, and raise and support his legs.

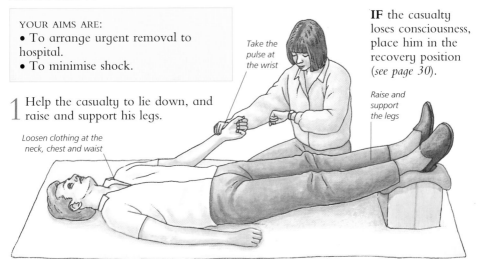

Take the pulse at the wrist

Raise and support the legs

Loosen clothing at the neck, chest and waist

2 Dial 999 for an ambulance. Insulate the casualty from cold. Check and record breathing, pulse, and level of response (*see page 50*) every 10 minutes.

3 Note the type, amount and source of any blood loss from body orifices (*see overleaf*). If possible, send a sample with the casualty to hospital.

BLEEDING FROM ORIFICES

Site	Appearance	Cause
Mouth	Bright red, frothy, coughed-up blood (*haemoptysis*). Vomited blood (*haematemesis*), possibly dark reddish-brown and resembling coffee grounds.	Bleeding in the lungs. Bleeding within the digestive system.
Ear	Fresh, bright-red blood. Thin, watery blood.	Injury to the inner ear; perforated ear drum. Leakage of cerebrospinal fluid following head injury.
Nose	Fresh, bright-red blood. Thin, watery blood.	Ruptured blood vessel in the nostril. Leakage of cerebrospinal fluid following head injury.
Anus	Fresh, bright-red blood. Black, tarry offensive-smelling stool (*melaena*).	Injury to the anus or lower bowel. Injury to the upper bowel.
Urethra	Urine with a red or smoky appearance (*haematuria*).	Bleeding from the bladder or kidneys.
Vagina	Either fresh or dark blood.	Menstruation; miscarriage; disease of, or injury to, the vagina or womb.

BLEEDING FROM THE EAR

Bleeding from inside the ear generally follows a rupture (*perforation*) of the ear-drum. Causes include a foreign body pushed into the ear, a blow to the side of the head, or an explosion. The casualty may experience a sharp pain as the ear-drum ruptures, followed by earache and deafness. If bleeding follows a head injury, the blood may appear thin and watery. This is very serious, as it indicates that fluid is leaking from around the brain.

See also: Foreign bodies in the ear, *page 177*. Head injuries, *page 117*.

TREATMENT

YOUR AIMS ARE:
- To allow blood to drain away.
- To minimise the risk of infection.

DO NOT plug the ear.

1 Help the casualty into a half-sitting position, with the head inclined to the injured side to let the blood drain.

2 Cover the ear with a sterile dressing or clean pad, lightly held in place.

3 Send or take the casualty to hospital in the treatment position.

NOSEBLEEDS

These most commonly occur when blood vessels inside the nostrils are ruptured, either by a blow to the nose, or as a result of sneezing, picking, or blowing the nose. Infection, such as a cold or 'flu, makes the blood vessels in the nose more fragile; nosebleeds may also occur as a result of high blood pressure. Nosebleeds are usually merely unpleasant, but they can sometimes be dangerous, since the casualty can lose a great deal of blood. Where a nosebleed follows a head injury, the blood may appear thin and watery. This is very serious, as it indicates that cerebrospinal fluid (*see page 114*) is leaking from around the brain.

See also: Head injuries, *page 117.*

TREATMENT

YOUR AIM IS:
• To control blood loss, and maintain an open airway.

1 Sit the casualty down with his head well forward. Don't let his head tip back; blood may run down the back of the throat, which can induce vomiting.

4 After 10 minutes, tell him to release the pressure. If the nose is still bleeding, reapply the pressure for further periods of 10 minutes.

IF the nosebleed persists beyond 30 minutes, take or send the casualty to hospital in the treatment position.

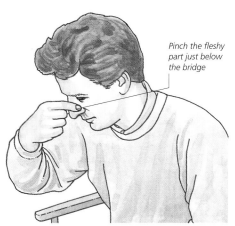

Pinch the fleshy part just below the bridge

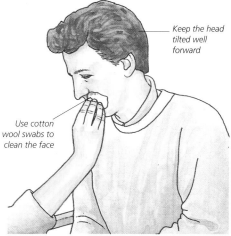

Keep the head tilted well forward

Use cotton wool swabs to clean the face

2 Ask the casualty to breathe through his mouth (this will also have a calming effect), and to pinch his nose just below the bridge. Help him if necessary.

3 Tell him to try not to speak, swallow, cough, spit, or sniff, as he may disturb blood clots. Give him a clean cloth or tissue to mop up dribble.

5 Once the bleeding is under control, and with the casualty still leaning forwards, gently clean around his nose and mouth with lukewarm water.

6 Advise the casualty to rest quietly for a few hours, and to avoid exertion and, in particular, blowing the nose, so as not to disturb the clot.

BLEEDING FROM THE MOUTH

Cuts to the tongue, lips, or lining of the mouth range from trivial injuries to more serious wounds. The cause is usually the casualty's own teeth, following a blow or fall. Bleeding may be profuse and appear alarming. Bleeding from a tooth socket may be the result of accidental loss of a tooth, or dental extraction.

TREATMENT

YOUR AIMS ARE:
- To control bleeding.
- To safeguard the airway by preventing the inhalation of blood.

1 Sit the casualty down, with her head forward and inclined towards the injured side, to allow blood to drain.

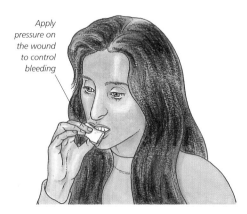

Apply pressure on the wound to control bleeding

2 To control the bleeding, place a gauze dressing pad over the wound and ask the casualty to squeeze it between her finger and thumb, maintaining the pressure for 10 minutes.

IF the bleeding is from a tooth socket, place a pad of gauze, thick enough to prevent the casualty's teeth from meeting when she bites, across the socket and tell her to bite on it.

3 If bleeding persists, replace the pad with a fresh one. Tell the casualty to let any escaping blood dribble; if swallowed, it may induce vomiting.

Knocked-out tooth
A knocked-out adult tooth may be successfully re-implanted in its socket. If it is lost, ask someone to look for it while you administer any necessary first aid.

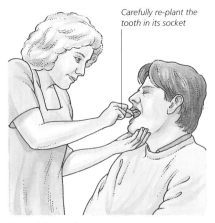

Carefully re-plant the tooth in its socket

Care of the tooth
Do not clean the tooth; you may damage the tissues that will regenerate. Replace the tooth in its socket, keeping it in position by pressing over a pad. Send or take the casualty to his dentist, or a hospital. If you cannot re-plant the tooth, store it in the casualty's cheek, or a cup of milk.

DO NOT wash the mouth out, as this may disturb a clot.

4 Advise the casualty to avoid hot drinks for 12 hours.

IF the wound is large, or if bleeding persists beyond 30 minutes or recurs, seek medical or dental advice.

VAGINAL BLEEDING

Bleeding from the vagina is most likely to be menstrual bleeding, which is often accompanied by abdominal cramps, but it can also indicate miscarriage, recent abortion, internal disease, or injury as a result of sexual assault. The history of the condition is essential to diagnosis, and has some bearing on first aid. If the bleeding is severe, shock may develop. Always be sensitive to a woman's feelings. She may be embarrassed, or may resent a male presence. Male First Aiders should, if possible, seek a female chaperone.

See also: Miscarriage, *page 190.*
Shock, *page 68.*

TREATMENT

> YOUR AIMS ARE:
> • To make the woman comfortable and reassure her.
> • To observe and treat for shock.
> • To arrange removal to hospital, if necessary.

1 Remove the woman, if possible, to a place with some privacy, or arrange for screening.

2 Give her a sanitary pad or a clean towel.

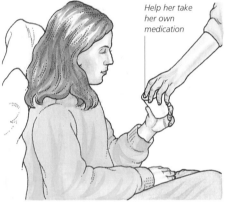

Help her take her own medication

IF she knows that any pains are menstrual cramps, she may take pain-killing tablets or drugs prescribed for their relief.

IF bleeding continues and is severe, dial 999 for an ambulance. Treat for shock.

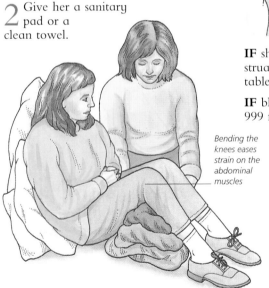

Bending the knees eases strain on the abdominal muscles

3 Make her comfortable, with her head and shoulders raised and supported, and her knees propped up.

Sexual assault

If a woman has been assaulted, it is vital not to disturb evidence by removing, washing, or disposing of clothing. Gently persuade her to refrain from washing herself and, if possible, from using the toilet until a forensic examination has been carried out by a specially trained doctor. It is important to note that a woman who has been assaulted may well feel threatened by a male "rescuer".

MAJOR WOUNDS

Many wounds, though very serious, do not cause severe external bleeding. This applies particularly to wounds to the trunk of the body; a stab wound to the abdomen, for example, may produce only a small, neat entry wound yet cause massive internal damage. Chest wounds can cause breathing complications; eye wounds can result in blindness.

PENETRATING CHEST WOUNDS

The heart and lungs, and the major blood vessels around them, lie within the chest (*thorax*), protected by the breastbone and the 12 pairs of ribs – the ribcage (*see page 136*). The ribcage also extends far enough to offer some protection to the upper abdominal organs.

A penetrating chest wound may thus cause severe internal damage within both chest and upper abdomen. The lungs are particularly vulnerable to injury, either directly, or because the wound perforates the membranes (*pleura*) that normally protect them. This allows air to enter the space between the membranes and exert pressure on the lung, which may cause it to collapse.

Sometimes pressure builds up to such an extent that it affects the uninjured lung. The pressure may also prevent adequate refilling of the heart, impairing the circulation and causing shock.

RECOGNITION

There will be:
• Difficult and painful breathing, possibly rapid, shallow, and uneven.
• An acute sense of alarm.

There may be:
• Signs of shock.
• Coughed-up frothy red blood.
• Blueness (*cyanosis*) at the mouth, nailbeds, and skin.
• A crackling feeling to the skin near the site of the wound, caused by air in the tissues.
• Blood bubbling out of the wound.
• In certain cases, the sound of air being sucked into the chest as the casualty breathes in.

See also: Shock, page 68.

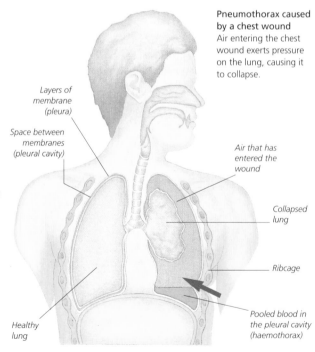

Pneumothorax caused by a chest wound
Air entering the chest wound exerts pressure on the lung, causing it to collapse.

Layers of membrane (pleura)

Space between membranes (pleural cavity)

Air that has entered the wound

Collapsed lung

Ribcage

Pooled blood in the pleural cavity (haemothorax)

Healthy lung

TREATMENT

YOUR AIMS ARE:
- To seal the wound and maintain breathing.
- To minimise shock.
- To arrange urgent removal to hospital.

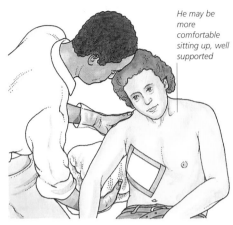

He may be more comfortable sitting up, well supported

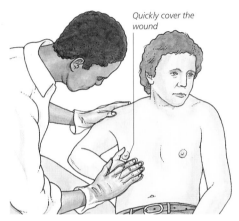

Quickly cover the wound

3 Support a conscious casualty in a comfortable position, inclined towards the injured side.

4 Dial 999 for an ambulance. Treat the casualty for shock if necessary.

1 Immediately use the palm of your hand or, if he is conscious, the casualty's hand, to cover the wound.

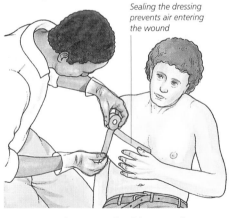

Sealing the dressing prevents air entering the wound

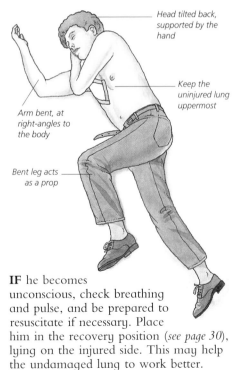

Head tilted back, supported by the hand

Keep the uninjured lung uppermost

Arm bent, at right-angles to the body

Bent leg acts as a prop

2 Cover the wound with a sterile dressing or clean pad, then cover the pad with a plastic bag, kitchen film, or foil, secured with adhesive strapping or firm bandaging to form an airtight seal.

IF he becomes unconscious, check breathing and pulse, and be prepared to resuscitate if necessary. Place him in the recovery position (*see page 30*), lying on the injured side. This may help the undamaged lung to work better.

ABDOMINAL WOUNDS

The severity of an abdominal wound may be evident in external bleeding and protruding abdominal contents. More commonly, there is hidden internal injury and bleeding. A stab wound, gunshot, or crushing injury to the abdomen may puncture, lacerate, or rupture organs and blood vessels deep within the body. The risk of infection is high.

See also: Internal bleeding, *page 83.*
Shock, *page 68.*

TREATMENT

YOUR AIMS ARE:
• To minimise the risk of infection.
• To minimise shock.

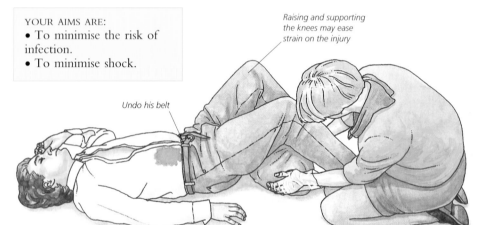

Raising and supporting the knees may ease strain on the injury

Undo his belt

1 Lay the casualty down, bending and supporting his knees if possible.

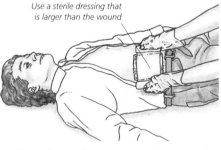

Use a sterile dressing that is larger than the wound

2 Put a large dressing over the wound, and secure it lightly in place with a bandage or adhesive strapping.

IF part of the intestine is protruding, do not touch it, but cover with a polythene bag or kitchen film to prevent it drying out. Alternatively, use a sterile dressing.

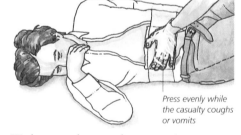

Press evenly while the casualty coughs or vomits

IF the casualty coughs or vomits, press firmly on the dressing to stop abdominal contents pushing through the wound.

3 Dial 999 for an ambulance. Treat the casualty for shock.

IF the casualty loses consciousness, check breathing and pulse, and be prepared to resuscitate if necessary. Place him in the recovery position (*see page 30*), supporting the abdomen as above.

EYE WOUNDS

The eye can be cut or bruised by direct blows or by sharp, chipped fragments of metal, grit, and glass. All eye injuries are potentially serious. Even superficial grazes to the surface (*cornea*) of the eye can lead to scarring or infection, with possible deterioration of vision.

A penetrating wound may rupture the eyeball and allow its clear fluid content (the *humour*) to escape. This type of injury is very serious, although it is now possible to repair eye wounds, and the sight in the eye may not be lost.

RECOGNITION

There will be:
- Intense pain in the affected eye, with spasm of the eyelids.

There may be:
- A visible wound.
- A bloodshot appearance to the injured eye, even if there is no visible wound.
- Partial or total loss of vision.
- Leakage of blood or clear fluid from a wound, possibly with flattening of the globe's normal round contour.

TREATMENT

> YOUR AIMS ARE:
> - To prevent further damage.
> - To arrange removal to hospital.

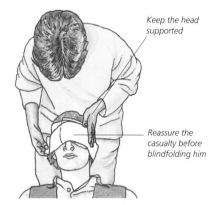

Keep the head supported

Reassure the casualty before blindfolding him

1 Lay the casualty on his back, holding his head to keep it as still as possible. Tell the casualty to keep both eyes still; movement of the "good" eye will cause movement of the injured one, which may damage it further.

DO NOT attempt to remove an embedded foreign body.

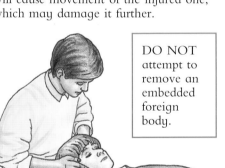

2 Cover the injured eye with an eyepad or sterile dressing, then, reassuring the casualty, bandage both eyes firmly enough to prevent movement.

3 Take or send the casualty to hospital in the treatment position.

Cradle the head to keep it still

CRUSH INJURIES

These are commonly caused by traffic accidents and incidents during building work, and by train crashes, explosions, earthquakes, or mining accidents.

Local injuries may include fractures, internal bleeding, blistering, and swelling. The crushing force may also impair the circulation, causing numbness at or below the site of injury; there may be no detectable pulse in a crushed limb.

The dangers of prolonged crushing

If the casualty is trapped for any length of time, there is the risk of two serious complications. First, prolonged crushing may cause extensive tissue damage, especially to muscles. Once the pressure is removed, shock may develop rapidly as tissue fluid leaks into the injured area.

Secondly, and more dangerously, toxic substances that have built up in muscles as a result of damage will be released suddenly into the circulation, and may cause kidney failure. This process, which is called "crush syndrome", is extremely serious and can be fatal.

See also: Fractures, *pages 141-142.*
Internal bleeding, *page 83.*
Shock, *page 68.*

TREATMENT

YOUR AIM IS:
• To obtain specialist medical aid urgently, taking any steps possible to treat the casualty meanwhile.

FOR A CASUALTY CRUSHED FOR LESS THAN 10 MINUTES

1 Release the casualty as quickly as possible.

2 Control any external bleeding and cover any wounds.

3 Secure and support any suspected fractures.

4 Examine and observe the casualty for signs of internal bleeding and shock, and treat accordingly.

5 Dial 999 for an ambulance. Make a note of the duration of crushing and the time of release.

FOR A CASUALTY CRUSHED FOR MORE THAN 10 MINUTES

DO NOT release the casualty.

1 Dial 999, giving clear details to the emergency services.

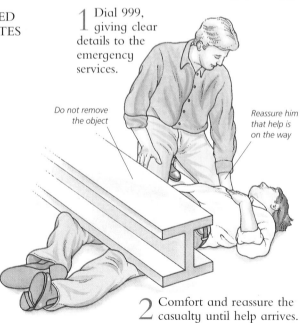

Do not remove the object

Reassure him that help is on the way

2 Comfort and reassure the casualty until help arrives.

AMPUTATION

The force and direction of an injury may be such that a limb, or part of a limb (for example, a finger or toe), is partially or completely severed. It is sometimes possible, using microsurgical techniques, to "re-plant" amputated parts. The sooner the casualty and severed part reach hospital the better. Describe the accident clearly to the emergency services; they will alert the specialist centre.

See also: Shock, *page 68.*

TREATMENT

YOUR AIMS ARE:
- To minimise blood loss and shock.
- To preserve the amputated part.

CARE OF THE CASUALTY

1 Control blood loss by applying direct pressure, and raising the injured part.

2 Apply a sterile dressing, or non-fluffy clean pad secured with a bandage.

3 Treat the casualty for shock.

4 Dial 999 for an ambulance, stating that the accident involves amputation. Accompany the casualty to hospital.

DO NOT use a tourniquet.

CARE OF THE AMPUTATED PART

1 Wrap the severed part in kitchen film or a polythene bag.

2 Wrap again in gauze or soft fabric, then place the package in another container (for example, another plastic bag) filled with crushed ice. Chilling will help preserve the part.

3 Mark the package with the time of injury and the casualty's name. Hand it over personally when help arrives.

DO NOT wash the severed part.

DO NOT apply cotton wool to any raw surface.

DO NOT allow the severed part to come into direct contact with ice.

IMPALEMENT

If someone becomes impaled by, for example, falling on railings, you must *never* attempt to lift him or her off; you may worsen internal injuries. Give clear details to the emergency services; they will bring specialist cutting equipment.

TREATMENT

YOUR AIM IS:
- To prevent further injury.

1 Dial 999 and explain the situation clearly. Send someone to make the call if possible.

2 Support the casualty's weight so that he or she is as comfortable as possible. Reassure the casualty constantly.

DO NOT give the casualty anything to eat or drink.

MINOR WOUNDS

Prompt first aid can help nature heal small wounds and deal with germs. But you must seek medical advice:
● If there is a foreign body embedded in the wound (*see opposite*).
● If the wound is at special risk of infection (such as a dog bite, or puncture by a dirty object).
● If a non-recent wound shows signs of becoming infected (*see page 96*).

Good wound care
● First wash your hands thoroughly.
● Avoid touching the wound with your fingers (use disposable gloves if possible).
● Don't talk, cough, or breathe over the wound or the dressing.
More details are given in *Dressings and Bandages (page 200)*, and in this book's companion volume, *Caring for the Sick*.

MINOR EXTERNAL BLEEDING

Minor bleeding is readily controlled by pressure and elevation. A small adhesive dressing is normally all that is necessary.

Medical aid need only be sought if the bleeding does not stop, or if the wound is at special risk of infection.

TREATMENT

YOUR AIM IS:
● To minimise the risk of infection.

1 Wash your hands thoroughly in soap and warm water.

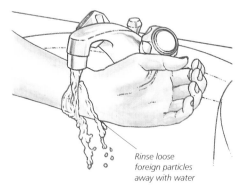

Rinse loose foreign particles away with water

2 If the wound is dirty, clean it by rinsing lightly under running water.

3 Pat gently dry with a sterile swab or clean tissue.

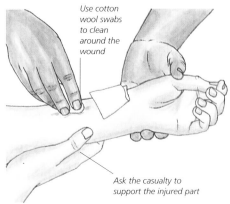

Use cotton wool swabs to clean around the wound

Ask the casualty to support the injured part

4 Temporarily cover the wound with sterile gauze. Clean the skin around it with soap and water (or a degreasing cleanser). Swab away from the wound and use a new swab for each stroke.

5 Pat dry, then cover the wound with an adhesive dressing (plaster).

IF there is a special risk of infection, advise the casualty to see her doctor.

FOREIGN BODIES IN MINOR WOUNDS

Small pieces of glass or grit lying on a wound can be carefully picked off, or rinsed off with cold water, before treatment. However, you must not try to remove objects that are embedded in the wound; you may cause further tissue damage and bleeding.

See also: Fish hooks, *page 175.*
  Splinters, *page 174.*

TREATMENT

> YOUR AIMS ARE:
> • To control bleeding without pressing the object into the wound.
> • To seek medical attention.

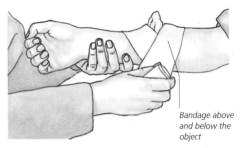

Bandage above and below the object

1 Control any bleeding by applying firm pressure on either side of the object, and raising the wounded part.

2 Drape a piece of gauze lightly over the wound to minimise the risk of germs entering it, then build up padding around the object until you can bandage without pressing down on it.

IF you cannot build the padding high enough, bandage around the object.

3 Take or send the casualty to hospital.

BRUISES

These are caused by internal bleeding that seeps through the tissues to produce discoloration under the skin. Bruising may develop very slowly and appear hours, even days, after injury. Bruising that develops rapidly and seems to be the main problem will benefit from first aid. Bruises may indicate deeper injury.

See also: Internal bleeding, *page 83.*

TREATMENT

> YOUR AIM IS:
> • To reduce blood flow to the injury, and minimise swelling, by means of cooling and compression.

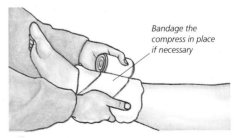

Bandage the compress in place if necessary

1 Raise and support the injured part in a comfortable position.

IF you suspect more serious underlying injury, such as a sprain or fracture, seek medical advice.

2 Apply a cold compress *(see page 203)* to the bruise.

INFECTION IN WOUNDS

All open wounds may be contaminated by micro-organisms (germs), either from the wounding source, from the air, or from the breath or fingers. Bleeding flushes some particles of dirt away; germs that remain may be destroyed naturally by the blood's white cells.

The dangers of infection

If dirt or dead tissue remain, there may be serious consequences. Germs can multiply and spread infection through the body (*septicaemia*), or tetanus infection (*see below*) may develop. Antibiotics or anti-tetanus injections may be needed for heavily contaminated or otherwise susceptible wounds. Wounds that show no signs of healing within 48 hours should also be considered infected. In these cases there may also be fever.

RECOGNITION

As infection develops, there may be:
• Increasing pain and soreness.
• Swelling, redness, and a feeling of heat around the injury.
• Pus within, or oozing from, the wound.
• Swelling and tenderness of the glands in the neck, armpit, or groin.
• Faint red trails on the skin of limbs leading to these glands.
• If the infection is advanced, signs of fever: sweating, thirst, shivering, and lethargy.

TREATMENT FOR AN INFECTED WOUND

YOUR AIMS ARE:
• To prevent further infection.
• To obtain medical aid.

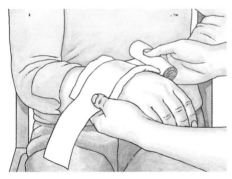

1 Cover the wound with a sterile dressing, or clean pad bandaged in place.

2 Raise and support the injured part to reduce swelling.

3 Tell the casualty to see his doctor. If the infection is advanced, call a doctor, or take or send him to hospital.

Tetanus

This is a dangerous infection that can develop if tetanus germs enter a wound. These germs are carried in the air and in soil as spores. When present in damaged and swollen tissues, they may release a poisonous substance (a *toxin*) that spreads through the nervous system, causing muscle spasms and paralysis.

Preventing tetanus

Tetanus is very difficult to treat, but can be prevented by immunisation, which is part of a baby's vaccination programme. Boosters are given on starting, and on leaving, school. Adults should receive further boosters every ten years.

Always ask a wounded casualty when he or she last had a tetanus injection. Seek medical advice:
• If the casualty has never been immunised.
• If the last injection was more than ten years ago.
• If the casualty cannot remember when the last injection was given.

BITES AND STINGS

A nimals and insects do not usually attack unless injured or otherwise provoked, and common sense can prevent many bites and stings. You must also take sensible precautions before attempting, for example, to rescue a casualty from an angry dog or a swarm of bees. If you cannot cope alone, get help or call the emergency services.

CONTENTS

When to seek medical attention

Though they can considerably mar a picnic or seaside excursion, insect and marine stings are often minor injuries, and first aid alone will generally suffice to relieve pain and discomfort.

Animal (and human) bites, however, always require some degree of medical attention, because germs are harboured in the mouths of all animals. Snake bites carry the additional risk of poisoning. Even if you have cleaned and dressed a bite wound satisfactorily, you must also ensure that the casualty is protected from such serious infections as tetanus and rabies.

THE FIRST AIDER SHOULD:

• Having ensured your own safety, remove the casualty from further danger.

• Treat any visible wound or painful symptoms, and minimise the risk of further injury and infection.

• Obtain medical attention if necessary.

• Note the time and nature of the injury, if possible identifying the attacking creature. This can enable medical personnel to deal with the injury itself and anticipate possible complications, or to establish the "trigger" for a severe allergic reaction.

ANIMAL BITES

Germs are harboured in the mouths of all animals (including humans). Bites from sharp, pointed teeth cause deep puncture wounds that carry germs far into the tissues. Human bites also crush the tissues. Hitting someone's teeth with a bare fist can produce a "bite" wound at the knuckles. Serious wounds require hospital care; any bite breaking the skin needs prompt first aid, followed by medical attention. These wounds are very vulnerable to infection.

See also: Minor wounds, *page 94.*
Severe external bleeding, *page 78.*
Tetanus, *page 96.*

TREATMENT

YOUR AIMS ARE:
• To control bleeding.
• To minimise the risk of infection, to the casualty and yourself.
• To obtain medical attention.

FOR SUPERFICIAL BITES

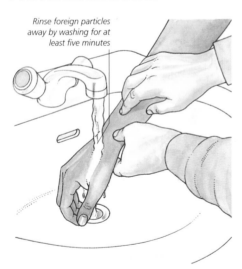

Rinse foreign particles away by washing for at least five minutes

1 Wash the wound thoroughly with soap and warm water.

2 Pat dry and cover with an adhesive dressing or a small sterile dressing.

3 Advise the casualty to see his own doctor.

Rabies

This is a potentially fatal viral infection of the nervous system, spread in the saliva of infected animals. Rabies is not currently found in the UK, but if a bite is sustained overseas, or from an animal that may have been smuggled into the UK, the casualty must receive anti-rabies injections. Rabies can only be confirmed if the animal is medically examined. Seek the help of the police to secure or retrieve a suspect animal.

FOR SERIOUS WOUNDS

1 Control bleeding by applying direct pressure and raising the injured part.

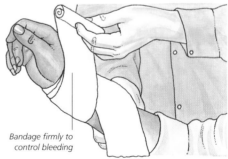

Bandage firmly to control bleeding

2 Cover the wound with a sterile dressing, or clean pad bandaged in place.

3 Take or send the casualty to hospital.

INSECT STINGS

Bee, wasp, and hornet stings are usually more painful and alarming than they are dangerous. An initial sharp pain is followed by mild swelling and soreness, which first aid can relieve. Some people, however, are allergic to these poisons, and can rapidly develop the serious condition, *anaphylactic shock*. Multiple stings can have a dangerous cumulative effect. Stings in the mouth or throat should be taken very seriously, as the swelling they cause can obstruct the airway.

See also: Anaphylactic shock, *page 71.*

TREATMENT

> YOUR AIMS ARE:
> • To relieve swelling and pain.
> • To arrange removal to hospital, if necessary.

FOR A STING IN THE SKIN

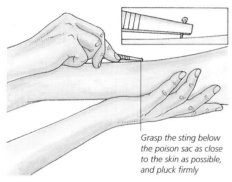

Grasp the sting below the poison sac as close to the skin as possible, and pluck firmly

1 Remove the sting, if it is still there, with tweezers.

2 Apply a cold compress (*see page 203*) to relieve pain and minimise swelling.

3 Advise the casualty to see her own doctor if pain and swelling persist or increase over the next day or two.

FOR A STING IN THE MOUTH

1 Give the casualty ice to suck, to minimise swelling.

2 Dial 999 for an ambulance. Reassure the casualty while waiting for help.

Tick bites

Ticks are tiny, spider-like creatures found in grass or woodland. They attach themselves to passing animals (including humans) and bite into the skin to suck blood. An unfed tick is very small and may not be noticed, particularly as its bite is painless; when sucking blood, it swells to the size of a pea and can easily be seen. Ticks can carry disease and cause infection, and should be removed as soon as possible. Once removed, put the tick in a container; the casualty must take it with him or her to a doctor.

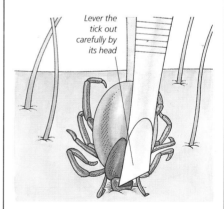

Lever the tick out carefully by its head

Removing a tick
Using fine-pointed tweezers, grasp the tick's head as close to the casualty's skin as possible. Use a slight to-and-fro action to lever, rather than pull, the head out. The mouthparts will be very firmly embedded in the skin; try to avoid breaking the tick and leaving the buried head behind.

INJURIES BY MARINE CREATURES

Sea creatures can cause injury in a number of ways. Stings can be caused by jellyfish and the related Portuguese man-of-war, corals, and sea anemones. Their venom is contained in stinging cells (*nematocysts*) that stick to the victim's skin. It is released when the cell ruptures.

If a spiny creature such as a sea urchin or weever fish is trodden on, its spines may puncture the skin and break off to become embedded in the foot. A painful local reaction will usually develop,

though serious general effects are rare. Most of the marine species normally encountered around the British Isles are not very toxic.

However, in some parts of the world, severe degrees of poisoning can occur with, rarely, fatal consequences resulting from a severe allergic reaction (anaphylactic shock), or paralysis of the chest muscle, which may cause drowning.

See also: Anaphylactic shock, *page 71.*

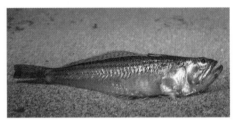

Weever fish
This fish, commonly found around Britain's coasts, lies buried in sand close to the shoreline, so is easily trodden on. Venomous spines on its gill covers and first dorsal fin may puncture the skin, causing swelling and soreness.

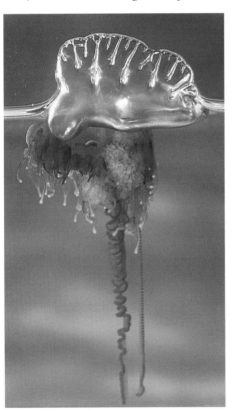

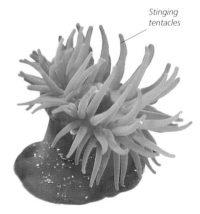

Stinging tentacles

Portuguese man-of-war
The name actually describes a jellyfish-like floating colony of creatures, with stinging tentacles that leave painful weals on the skin. The venom is rarely fatal, but multiple stings may cause complications.

Sea anemone
These small creatures are most commonly encountered in rock pools. If touched or trodden on, venomous stinging cells on their tentacles, or ejected from the anemone's "mouth", may cause great pain.

TREATMENT FOR MARINE STINGS

YOUR AIMS ARE:
- To reassure the casualty.
- To inactivate stinging cells before they release their venom, and neutralise any free venom.
- To relieve pain and discomfort.

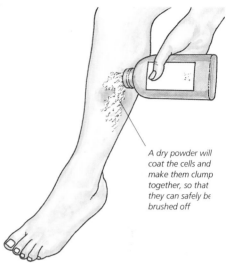

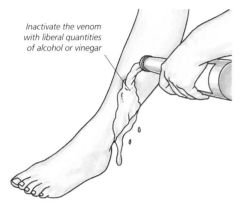

Inactivate the venom with liberal quantities of alcohol or vinegar

A dry powder will coat the cells and make them clump together, so that they can safely be brushed off

1 Pour alcohol (any alcoholic drink will do) or household vinegar over the injury for a few minutes to incapacitate stinging cells that have not yet fired.

2 Apply a paste of equal parts of sodium bicarbonate (baking soda) and water to the wound.

3 Dust a dry powder over the skin around the injury to make remaining cells stick together. Talcum powder will suffice — better still is meat tenderiser, used in barbecue cooking; papain, one of its ingredients, can inactivate venom.

IF the injuries are severe, or there is a serious generalised reaction, dial 999 for an ambulance. If the casualty is having difficulty breathing, she may be in anaphylactic shock; treat as on page 71.

TREATMENT FOR MARINE PUNCTURE WOUNDS

YOUR AIMS ARE:
- To inactivate the venom.
- To obtain medical aid.

1 Put the injured part in water as hot as the casualty can bear for at least 30 minutes. Top up the water as it cools, being careful not to scald the casualty.

2 Take or send the casualty to hospital, where spines remaining in the skin may have to be removed.

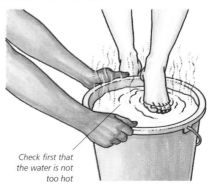

Check first that the water is not too hot

SNAKE BITES

The only poisonous snake native to the United Kingdom is the adder, whose bite is rarely fatal. However, more exotic snakes are kept as pets. While a snake bite is often not a serious injury, it can be very frightening. Reassurance is vital, for if the casualty keeps still and calm, the spread of venom may be delayed.

Keep the snake, or record its appearance, so that, if necessary, the right anti-venom can be given. Notify the police if an escaped snake remains at large.

RECOGNITION

Depending on the species, there may be:

• A pair of puncture marks.
• Severe pain at the site of the bite.
• Redness and marked swelling around the bite.
• Nausea and vomiting.
• Laboured breathing; in extreme cases, breathing may stop altogether.
• Disturbed vision.
• Increased salivation and sweating.

TREATMENT

YOUR AIMS ARE:
• To reassure the casualty.
• To prevent the spread of venom through the body.
• To arrange urgent removal to hospital.

1 Lay the casualty down. Tell her to keep calm and still.

2 Wash the wound thoroughly with soap and water, if available.

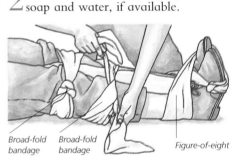

Broad-fold bandage   Broad-fold bandage   Figure-of-eight

3 Secure and support the injured part. Dial 999 for an ambulance.

DO NOT apply a tourniquet, slash at the wound with a knife, or attempt to suck out the venom.

Keep the wounded part below the level of the heart, so that the venom is contained locally

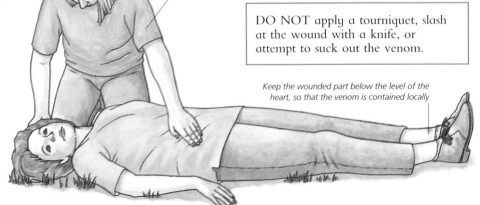

Reassure the casualty constantly

BURNS AND SCALDS

B urns result from dry heat, from corrosive substances, and from friction; scalds are caused by
wet heat – hot liquids and vapours. Burns can also
be produced by extreme cold, and by radiation,
including the sun's rays.

Burns may be incidental to, or a consequence
of, situations that pose a greater threat to life.
Fires may be started accidentally by victims of
drug or alcohol overdose, or there may be other
serious injuries caused by an explosion, or a jump
from a burning building. Once burns are treated,
the casualty should be thoroughly examined.

Dealing with a burns incident

The approach to an accident resulting in burns is
frequently complicated by the presence of fire,
explosions, electrical danger, toxic fumes, or other
hazards (see Action at an Emergency, pages 13-24).
Burns can be very frightening, particularly when a
flame burn occurs in an enclosed space. Both you
and the casualty may be distressed by the smell of
singed hair and burned flesh.

CONTENTS

THE FIRST AIDER SHOULD:

• Establish your own safety *before* attempting to
treat the casualty.

• Stop the burning, by means of rapid cooling, in
order to prevent further damage to the tissues, to
reduce swelling, minimise shock, and alleviate pain.

• Cover the injury. Burns are extremely susceptible
to infection, so they need protection from germs.

• Except in the case of very minor burns, obtain
appropriate medical aid.

ASSESSING A BURN

There are a number of factors to consider when assessing the severity of a burn and how best to treat it. These include the cause of the burn, whether the airway is involved (*see right*), the depth of the burn, and its extent.

The extent of the burn will tell you whether shock (*see page 68*) is likely to develop, as tissue fluid (*serum*) leaks from the burned area and is replenished by fluids from the circulatory system. The greater the area covered by the burn, the more severe shock will be. The cause of the burn may also alert you to any other possible complications.

Burns also carry a serious risk of infection, and the larger and deeper the burn, the greater this risk will be. The damage to the skin caused by burning breaks down the body's natural barrier, leaving it exposed to germs.

Airway involvement in burns

Any part of the air passages may be damaged by toxic smoke, hot gases or corrosive chemicals. These are serious injuries. The tissues may swell rapidly, making breathing very difficult.

Recognition

Suspect that the airway is at risk when a burn has been sustained in a confined space, or if you notice:
- Soot around the nose or mouth.
- Singeing of the nasal hairs.
- Redness, swelling, or actual burning of the tongue.
- Damaged skin around the mouth.
- Hoarseness of the voice.
- Breathing difficulty.

Whatever the cause or extent, burns involving a casualty's airway always require immediate hospital treatment.

HOW BURNS ARE CAUSED

Type of burn	Causes
Dry burn	Flames • Contact with hot objects, for example, domestic appliances, or cigarettes • Friction, for example rope burns
Scald	Steam • Hot liquids such as tea and coffee, or hot fat
Electrical burn	Low-voltage current, as used by domestic appliances • Arcing from high-voltage currents • Lightning strikes
Cold injury	Frostbite • Contact with freezing metals • Contact with freezing vapours, such as liquid oxygen or liquid nitrogen
Chemical burn	Industrial chemicals, including inhaled fumes and corrosive gases Domestic chemicals and agents, such as paint stripper, caustic soda, weedkillers, bleach, oven cleaner, or any other strong acid or alkali
Radiation burn	Sunburn • Over-exposure to ultra-violet lamp ("sunlamp") • Exposure to radioactive source

DEPTH OF BURNS

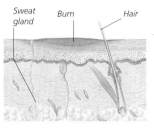

Sweat gland | Burn | Hair

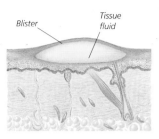

Blister | Tissue fluid

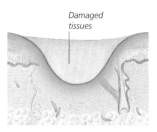

Damaged tissues

Superficial burns
These involve only the outer layer of the skin, and are characterised by redness, swelling, and tenderness. Classic examples are mild sunburn, or a scald produced by a splash of hot tea or coffee. Superficial burns usually heal well if prompt first aid is given, and do not require medical attention unless extensive.

Partial-thickness burns
A burn damaging a "partial thickness" of the skin requires medical treatment. The skin will look raw, and blisters will form. These burns usually heal well, but, if extensive, they can be serious; partial-thickness burns affecting more than 50 per cent of the body's surface (less in children and the elderly) can be fatal.

Full-thickness burns
In "full-thickness" burns, all layers of the skin are burned. Damage may extend beyond the skin to affect nerves, muscle, and fat. The skin may appear pale, waxy, and sometimes charred. Full-thickness burns of any size always need medical attention without delay, and will usually require specialist treatment.

EXTENT OF BURNS

The area of a burn gives an approximate indication of the degree of shock that will develop, and, with depth, can be used as a guide to the level of treatment required.

Extent is expressed in terms of a percentage of the body's total surface area. The "rules of nine", which divide the surface area of the body into areas of approximately nine per cent, are used to calculate extent and to decide what level of medical attention should be sought. For an otherwise healthy adult:
• Any partial-thickness burn of one per cent or more (covering an area approximating to that of the casualty's hand) must be seen by a doctor.
• A partial-thickness burn of nine per cent or more will cause shock to develop; the casualty needs hospital treatment.
• A full-thickness burn of any size requires hospital treatment.

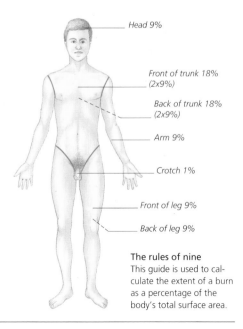

Head 9%
Front of trunk 18% (2x9%)
Back of trunk 18% (2x9%)
Arm 9%
Crotch 1%
Front of leg 9%
Back of leg 9%

The rules of nine
This guide is used to calculate the extent of a burn as a percentage of the body's total surface area.

SEVERE BURNS AND SCALDS

Depth, extent, and, possibly, circumstances will swiftly alert you to a burn's severity. The priority is to cool the injury; the longer the burning is allowed to go unchecked, the more severely the casualty will be injured.

Follow the ABC of resuscitation only once cooling is under way. Remember, too, that all severe burns carry with them the danger of shock.

See also: Fires, *page 20*
Shock, *page 68.*

TREATMENT

> YOUR AIMS ARE:
> • To halt the burning process and relieve pain.
> • To resuscitate if necessary.
> • To treat associated injuries.
> • To minimise the risk of infection.
> • To arrange urgent removal to hospital.

> DO NOT overcool the casualty; this treatment carries with it the risk of dangerously lowering the body temperature (*hypothermia*).
>
> DO NOT remove anything sticking to the burn; you may cause further damage and introduce infection.

1 Lay the casualty down, if possible protecting the burned area from contact with the ground.

2 Douse the burn with copious amounts of cold liquid. Thorough cooling may take 10 minutes or more, but this must not delay the casualty's removal to hospital.

3 While cooling the burn, check airway, breathing, and pulse, and be prepared to resuscitate if necessary.

4 Gently remove any rings, watches, belts, shoes, or smouldering clothing from the injured area, before it begins to swell. Carefully remove burned clothing unless it is sticking to the burn.

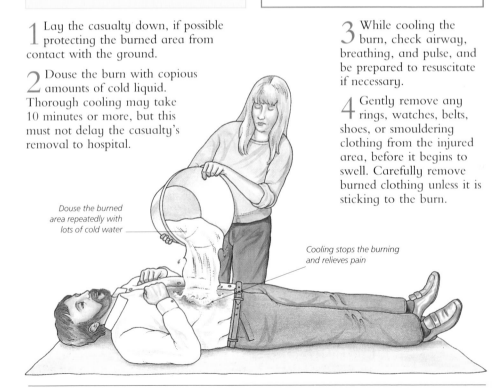

Douse the burned area repeatedly with lots of cold water

Cooling stops the burning and relieves pain

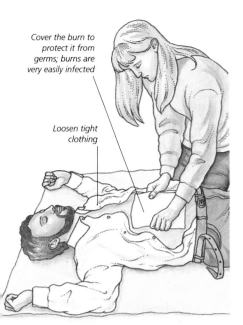

Cover the burn to protect it from germs; burns are very easily infected

Loosen tight clothing

Dressing a burn

All burns should be covered to protect them from infection, though the dressing does not need to be secured unless on an awkward part of the body. Use a burns sheet if possible, or improvise with clean, *non-fluffy* material, such as:
- A portion of a freshly-laundered sheet or pillowcase.
- Plastic kitchen film. Discard the first two turns from the roll.
- A clean plastic bag for a burned hand or foot. Secure it with a bandage or strapping, over the plastic, not the skin.

DO NOT touch or otherwise interfere with the injured area.

DO NOT burst any blisters.

DO NOT apply lotions, ointment, or fat to the injury.

5 Cover the injury with a sterile burns sheet or other suitable material (*see box*). (Burns to the face do not need to be covered. Keep cooling them with water to relieve the pain.)

6 Ensure that an ambulance is on its way. While waiting, treat the casualty for shock. Monitor and record breathing and pulse, and be prepared to resuscitate if necessary.

BURNS TO THE MOUTH AND THROAT

Burns to the face and burns within the mouth or throat are very dangerous, as they cause rapid swelling and inflammation of the air passages. Usually, signs of burning will be evident (*see page 104*).

There is no specific first aid treatment for an extreme case; the swelling will rapidly block the airway, and there is a serious risk of suffocation. Immediate and highly specialised medical aid is required.

TREATMENT

YOUR AIM IS:
- To obtain specialist medical aid as quickly as possible.

1 Dial 999 for an ambulance. Tell the control officer that you suspect burns to the airway.

2 Take any steps possible to improve the casualty's air supply; for example, loosening clothing around the neck. Give oxygen if you are trained to do so.

IF the casualty becomes unconscious, place in the recovery position (*see page 30*). Be prepared to attempt resuscitation.

MINOR BURNS AND SCALDS

Domestic accidents are the most common cause of minor burns and scalds. Prompt first aid will usually enable them to heal naturally and well, but if you are in any doubt as to the severity of the injury, seek a doctor's advice.

TREATMENT

YOUR AIMS ARE:
- To stop the burning.
- To relieve pain and swelling.
- To minimise the risk of infection.

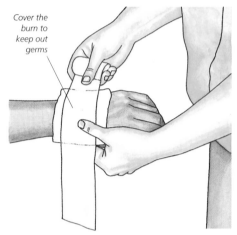

Cover the burn to keep out germs

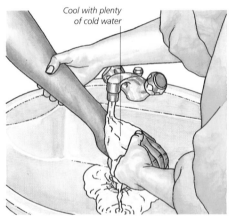

Cool with plenty of cold water

3 Cover the area with a sterile dressing, or any clean, non-fluffy material. A polythene bag or kitchen film makes a good temporary covering.

1 Flood the injured part with cold water for about 10 minutes to stop the burning and relieve the pain. If water is unavailable, any cold, harmless liquid, such as milk or canned drinks, will do.

2 Gently remove any jewellery, watches, or constricting clothing from the injured area before it begins to swell.

DO NOT use adhesive dressings or strapping.

DO NOT break blisters or interfere with the injured area.

DO NOT apply lotions, ointments, creams, or fats to the injury.

Blisters

These are thin "bubbles" that form on skin damaged by heat or friction. They are the result of tissue fluid (*serum*) leaking into the burned area below the skin's surface. During healing, new skin forms at the base of the blister; the serum is absorbed and the outer layer of dead skin eventually peels off.

What you can do
Never break a blister; you are likely to introduce infection. A blister usually needs no treatment. However, if it breaks, or is likely to be damaged, cover the injured area with a dry, non-adherent dressing that extends well beyond the blister's edges.

SPECIAL TYPES OF BURN

Many burns are caused not by direct heat, but by heat produced within the body tissues by, for example, strong chemicals or electricity. The type of damage caused is, however, the same as that produced by "thermal" burns, and first aid follows the same guidelines. With accidents involving high-voltage electricity or harmful chemicals, remember that your first priority is your own safety. You must not endanger yourself or others by treating a casualty in hazardous circumstances, however urgent the casualty's needs appear.

See also: Action at an Emergency, *pages 13-24.*

ELECTRICAL BURNS

Burns may occur when electricity passes through the body. Much of the visible damage occurs at the points of entry and exit of the current. However, there may also be a track of internal damage.

How electrical burns are caused

Burns may be caused by a lightning strike, or by low- or high-voltage current. An electric shock can cause cardiac arrest; if the casualty is unconscious, your immediate priority is thus the ABC of resuscitation. The position and direction of entry and exit wounds will alert you to the likely extent of hidden injury, and to the degree of shock that may ensue.

RECOGNITION

There may be:
- Unconsciousness.
- Full-thickness burns, with swelling, scorching, and charring, at both the point of entry and exit.
- If the casualty has been a victim of "arcing" high-voltage electricity, a brown, coppery residue on the skin. (Do not mistake this for injury.)
- Signs of shock.

See also: Electrical injuries, *page 22.*
Severe burns and scalds, *page 106.*
Shock, *page 68.*
Unconsciousness, *page 116.*

TREATMENT

YOUR AIMS ARE:
- To treat the burns and shock.
- To arrange urgent removal to hospital.

DO NOT approach a victim of high-voltage electricity until you are officially informed that the current has been switched off and isolated.

IF the casualty is unconscious, immediately open the airway, check breathing and pulse, and be prepared to resuscitate if necessary.

1 Flood the site(s) of injury with cold water, as described on page 106.

2 Place a sterile burns sheet, sterile dressing, or other clean, non-fluffy material over the burn(s).

3 Dial 999 for an ambulance. Treat the casualty for shock.

CHEMICAL BURNS

Certain chemicals may irritate or damage the skin, or be absorbed through the skin, causing widespread and some-times fatal damage within the body. Unlike thermal burns, the signs of chemical burns develop slowly. The principles of first aid are, however, the same.

Most strong corrosives are found in industry, though chemical burns can also be caused by domestic agents such as oven cleaners and paint stripper. These injuries are always serious, and may require urgent hospital treatment. It may be helpful to discover and note the name, or brand name, of the substance. Ensure your own safety when approaching and treating these injuries; note that some chemicals give off deadly fumes.

RECOGNITION

There may be:
• Intense, stinging pain.
• At first, little to see, then redness or staining, and blistering and peeling.

See also: Inhalation of fumes, *page 60.*
Hazchem symbols, *page 19.*
Industrial poisons, *page 169.*

TREATMENT

YOUR AIMS ARE:
• To identify and remove the chemical before it can do more harm.
• To arrange removal to hospital.

DO NOT delay starting treatment by searching for an antidote.

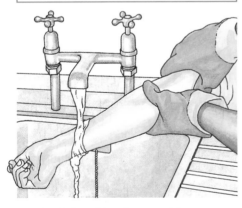

1 Flood the affected area with water to disperse the chemical and stop the burning process. Irrigate for longer than you would for a thermal burn; some chemicals may need 20 minutes.

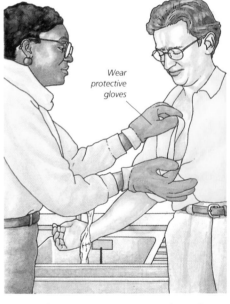

Wear protective gloves

2 Gently remove any contaminated clothing while flooding the injury. Be sure not to contaminate yourself – use protective gloves if available.

3 Take or send the casualty to hospital, keeping a close watch on airway and breathing.

CHEMICAL BURNS TO THE EYE

Splashes of chemicals in the eye can cause serious injury if not treated quickly. They can damage the surface of the eye, resulting in scarring and even blindness. Be especially careful, while irrigating the eye, that contaminated rinsing water does not splash you or the casualty. Wear protective gloves if they are available.

RECOGNITION

There may be:

- Intense pain in the eye.
- Inability to open the injured eye.
- Redness and swelling in and around the eye.
- Copious watering of the eye.

TREATMENT

> YOUR AIMS ARE:
> - To disperse the harmful chemical.
> - To arrange removal to hospital.

> DO NOT allow the casualty to rub or touch the eye.

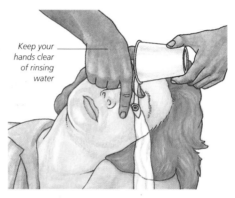

Keep your hands clear of rinsing water

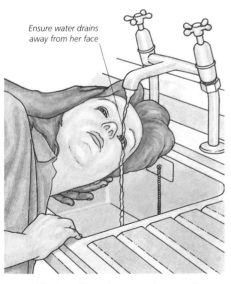

Ensure water drains away from her face

2 If the eye is shut in a spasm of pain, gently but firmly pull the eyelids open. Be careful that contaminated water does not splash the sound eye.

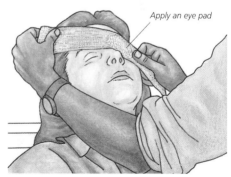

Apply an eye pad

1 Hold the affected eye under gently running cold water for at least 10 minutes. Make sure you irrigate both sides of the eyelid thoroughly. You may find it easier to pour the water from an eye irrigator or a glass.

3 Cover the eye with a sterile eye pad or pad of clean, non-fluffy material.

4 Take or send the casualty to hospital.

SUNBURN

This can be caused by over-exposure to the rays of the sun or a sunlamp. Similar burns can also, rarely, be caused by exposure to a radioactive source. Most are superficial burns, with redness, itching, and tenderness. In severe cases, the skin is lobster-red and blistered; the casualty may also suffer heatstroke.

Occasionally, exaggerated reactions to sun exposure can be precipitated by the use of some medicines. At high altitudes, sunburn can occur even on a dull, overcast day in summer (from "skyshine"), or by reflection from snow in winter.

See also: Heatstroke, *page 134.*

TREATMENT

YOUR AIMS ARE:
- To move the casualty out of the sun and into a cool place.
- To relieve discomfort and pain.

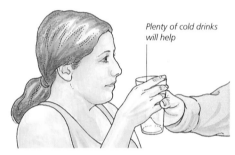

Plenty of cold drinks will help

1 Help the casualty into the shade or, preferably, indoors.

2 Cool her skin by sponging with cold water, or soaking in a cold bath.

IF there is extensive blistering or other skin damage, seek medical advice.

3 Give her frequent sips of cold water. If the burns are mild, calamine or an after-sun preparation may soothe them.

FLASH BURNS TO THE EYE

If the eyes are exposed to prolonged glare produced by the reflection of the sun's rays from a bright surface, such as snow or concrete, the surface (*cornea*) of the eye may be damaged. This painful condition, which may take as long as a week to subside, can also be caused by ultra-violet light. When caused by a welding torch, the condition is known as "welder's flash" or "arc eye".

RECOGNITION

The symptoms and signs do not usually appear for some time after exposure.
There will be:
- Intense pain in the affected eye(s).
There may be:
- A "gritty" feeling in the eye(s).
- Sensitivity to light.
- Redness and watering of the eye(s).

TREATMENT

YOUR AIMS ARE:
- To prevent further damage.
- To obtain medical attention.

1 Apply and secure eye pads. Reassure the casualty before covering the eyes.

2 Take or send the casualty to hospital.

DISORDERS OF CONSCIOUSNESS

A fully conscious person is awake, alert, and aware of his or her surroundings. Whereas sleep is a normal state of lowered consciousness, unconsciousness is an abnormal state that disables the body's reflexes. When a person is asleep, vital functions such as breathing take place automatically; if the person is unconscious and lying on his or her back, the tongue may fall to the back of the throat and block the airway. Any unconscious casualty may therefore require immediate first aid.

What you will find in this chapter

This chapter covers first aid for unconsciousness caused by physical damage to the brain (such as head injury), or by interference with the brain's blood supply (for example, a stroke). In addition, there are techniques to manage and treat episodes of impaired consciousness, caused by conditions such as epilepsy that disrupt the nervous system.

CONTENTS

THE FIRST AIDER SHOULD:

• Open an unconscious casualty's airway to ensure that he or she can breathe. Check airway, breathing, and circulation every few minutes. Make a record of the pulse and breathing rate.

• Protect a casualty whose consciousness is impaired from harm.

• Monitor and record the casualty's level of response. This may help medical decisions about treatment.

• Look for, and treat, associated injuries.

• Arrange urgent removal to hospital if unconsciousness persists beyond three minutes, or if you suspect a serious condition such as skull fracture or stroke.

THE NERVOUS SYSTEM

The nervous system comprises the brain, the spinal cord, and the nerves. Its function is to carry signals to and from all parts of the body, registering and acting on stimuli, regulating bodily functions, and controlling all movement. Most muscle action is controlled by the will, but the vital functions of the body, such as the circulation, respiration, and digestion, are regulated by the autonomic nervous system, a complex network controlled by centres in the brain stem that operate independently of the level of consciousness.

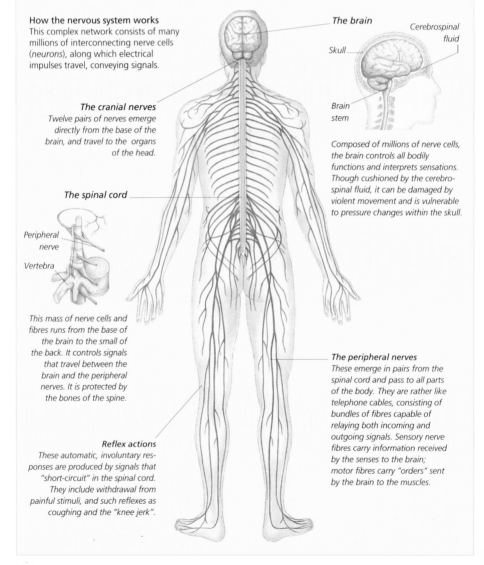

How the nervous system works
This complex network consists of many millions of interconnecting nerve cells (*neurons*), along which electrical impulses travel, conveying signals.

The cranial nerves
Twelve pairs of nerves emerge directly from the base of the brain, and travel to the organs of the head.

The spinal cord

Peripheral nerve

Vertebra

This mass of nerve cells and fibres runs from the base of the brain to the small of the back. It controls signals that travel between the brain and the peripheral nerves. It is protected by the bones of the spine.

Reflex actions
These automatic, involuntary responses are produced by signals that "short-circuit" in the spinal cord. They include withdrawal from painful stimuli, and such reflexes as coughing and the "knee jerk".

The brain

Cerebrospinal fluid

Skull

Brain stem

Composed of millions of nerve cells, the brain controls all bodily functions and interprets sensations. Though cushioned by the cerebrospinal fluid, it can be damaged by violent movement and is vulnerable to pressure changes within the skull.

The peripheral nerves
These emerge in pairs from the spinal cord and pass to all parts of the body. They are rather like telephone cables, consisting of bundles of fibres capable of relaying both incoming and outgoing signals. Sensory nerve fibres carry information received by the senses to the brain; motor fibres carry "orders" sent by the brain to the muscles.

UNCONSCIOUSNESS

This is an abnormal state resulting from an interruption of the brain's normal activity. Whatever the cause, there are three rules of treatment you must follow.

• *Ensure that the airway is open and clear*
Any unconscious casualty's airway is in constant danger, particularly if he or she is lying face-up. The tongue may flop to the back of the throat, and muscles that normally keep the airway open lose their control. There is no cough reflex to clear saliva from the throat. Stomach contents may be regurgitated and inhaled.

• *Check and re-check the level of response*
Short of full unconsciousness (*coma*) there are many degrees of impairment of awareness and response. To make a

rapid initial assessment of responsiveness, use the "AVPU" aide-memoire:

A - **A**lert
V - responds to **V**oice
P - responds to **P**ain
U - **U**nresponsive

A more detailed assessment can be made, and should be repeated every 10 minutes, using the simplified version, *below*, of the Glasgow Coma Scale (as used in hospitals). This checklist forms part of the observation chart on page 50.

• *Examine the casualty thoroughly*
Impaired consciousness can mask other injuries, so thorough examination is vital. Both the casualty's condition and level of response may alter with time.

MAJOR CAUSES OF UNCONSCIOUSNESS

Condition	Cause
Direct damage to the brain	Head injury
Interference with blood supply to the brain	Stroke • Fainting • Heart attack • Shock
Compression of the brain	Head injury • Stroke • Some infections • Some tumours
Disturbance of chemical content of blood supplied to the brain	Low blood oxygen (*hypoxia*) • Poisoning, including alcohol and drug intoxication • Low blood sugar (*hypoglycaemia*)
Other conditions	Epilepsy • Abnormal body temperature

ASSESSING THE LEVEL OF RESPONSE

Eyes – do they:	Speech – does the casualty:	Movement – does the casualty:
• Open spontaneously? • Open on command? • Open to a painful stimulus? • Remain closed?	• Respond sensibly to questions? • Appear confused? • Make incomprehensible sounds? • Make no response?	• Obey commands? • Move in response to a painful stimulus? • Make no response?

EXAMINING AND TREATING AN UNCONSCIOUS CASUALTY

YOUR AIMS ARE:
- To maintain an open airway.
- To assess and record the level of response.
- To treat any associated injuries.
- To arrange, if necessary, urgent removal to hospital.

3 Control any bleeding (*see page 78*) and support suspected fractures (*see pages 141-142*). As you work, look for less obvious injury or conditions. Smell her breath, and look for needle marks. Look for warning bracelets, lockets or cards. Ask bystanders for information.

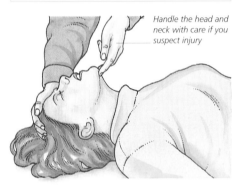

Handle the head and neck with care if you suspect injury

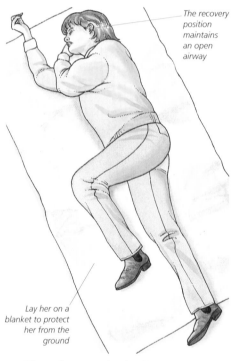

The recovery position maintains an open airway

Lay her on a blanket to protect her from the ground

1 Open the airway by lifting the chin and tilting the head. Check breathing and pulse, and be prepared to resuscitate if necessary. Check and record the casualty's level of response (*see previous page*).

IF she starts to vomit, immediately place her in the recovery position (*see page 30*).

2 Examine the casualty quickly but systematically to identify any severe external bleeding or major fractures.
- Try to avoid stepping over an unconscious casualty.

DO NOT try to give an unconscious casualty anything by mouth.

DO NOT move the casualty unnecessarily, because of the possibility of spinal injury. Never attempt to make an unconscious person sit or stand upright.

DO NOT leave an unconscious casualty unattended.

4 Place the casualty in the recovery position (*see page 30*).

IF the casualty does not regain full consciousness within 3 minutes, dial 999 for an ambulance. Record breathing and pulse rate, and level of response, every 10 minutes, using the observation chart on page 50. Send the chart with the casualty to hospital.

IF the casualty regains full consciousness within 3 minutes, and remains well after a further 10 minutes, advise her to see her doctor.

HEAD INJURIES

All injuries to the head are potentially dangerous, and always need medical attention, particularly if severe enough to cause impaired consciousness. This may indicate damage to the brain, damage to blood vessels inside the skull, or skull fracture. Any head injury may also cause injury to the spine, which must be protected. A scalp wound (*see page 80*) may be present but there may be no visible evidence of underlying damage. Impaired consciousness may mask the presence of other injuries: examine the casualty closely. Although unconsciousness may result from a head injury, the injury may be the result of falling unconscious from another cause.

CONCUSSION

The brain is free to move a little within the skull, and can thus be "shaken" by a violent blow. This may cause concussion, a condition of widespread but, usually, temporary disturbance of the brain. The period of unconsciousness is always brief and is always followed by complete recovery – by definition, concussion can only be safely diagnosed once the casualty has fully recovered.

RECOGNITION

There will be:

• Brief or partial loss of consciousness following a blow to the head.

There may be:

• Dizziness or nausea on recovery.
• Loss of memory of events at the time of, or immediately preceding, the injury.
• A mild, generalised headache.

See also: Unconsciousness, page 115.

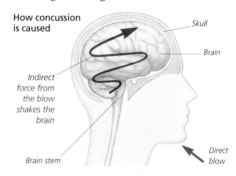

How concussion is caused

Skull

Brain

Indirect force from the blow shakes the brain

Brain stem

Direct blow

TREATMENT

YOUR AIMS ARE:
• To maintain an open airway and adequate breathing.
• If necessary, to seek medical aid.

1 Place the casualty in the recovery position (*see page 30*). Monitor and record breathing, pulse, and level of response (*page 50*). If the casualty remains unconscious after three minutes, dial 999 for an ambulance. If the casualty swiftly regains consciousness, watch closely for any deterioration in the level of response, even after an apparent full recovery.

2 Place the casualty in the care of a responsible person. Do not allow a casualty injured on the sports field to "play on" without a doctor's approval.

3 Advise the casualty to see his or her own doctor.

SKULL FRACTURE

The skull is a domed vault with an irregular and complex base. It surrounds and protects the brain. Fractures of the skull are thus potentially very serious injuries, because there may be associated brain damage. Sometimes this is merely concussion (*see page 117*); more seriously, the brain can be bruised (*cerebral contusion*), or there may be bleeding within the skull that accumulates and exerts pressure on the brain (*cerebral compression*).

When to suspect skull fracture

A wound may alert you to the possibility of fracture, and also presents the danger that germs, and hence infection, can enter the brain. There may be cerebrospinal fluid leaking from the ear or nose, as clear fluid or watery blood. This is not only a serious sign, but also indicates another entry point for germs.

Suspect a fractured skull in any casualty who has received a head injury resulting in unconsciousness. Note,

however, that it is violent head movement (especially "fore-and-aft") that causes unconsciousness. Some injuries (for example, crushing) can fracture the skull without causing loss of consciousness.

RECOGNITION

Any of the following may be present:
● A wound or bruise on the head.
● A soft, boggy area or depression of the scalp.
● Impairment of consciousness.
● A progressive deterioration in the level of response.
● A flow of clear fluid or watery blood from the nose or ear.
● Blood in the white of the eye.
● Distortion or lack of symmetry of the head or face.

See also: Back injuries, *page 153.*
Bleeding from the scalp, *page 80.*
Unconsciousness, *page 115.*

Causes of skull fracture

The skull may be fractured in several different ways, by both direct force (a blow to the head) and indirect force (for example, a fall from a height, landing heavily on the feet). Fractures caused by indirect force commonly occur at the base of the skull, and these injuries may be accompanied by damage to the spinal column (*see page 153*).

Types of fracture

Many types of skull fracture, particularly linear fractures (cracks) in the domed vault and fractures to the base of the skull, can only be diagnosed by X-ray or other imaging methods in hospital. Severe injuries may cause multiple cracking (an "eggshell" fracture), which may extend to the base of the skull. A "depressed" fracture may cause bone fragments to be driven in to injure, and exert damaging pressure on, the brain.

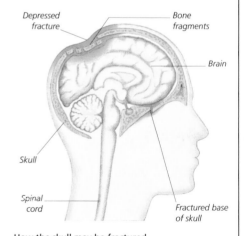

How the skull may be fractured
A depressed fracture is caused by a direct blow; a fracture of the base of the skull may be caused by landing heavily on the feet or the base of the spine.

TREATMENT

YOUR AIMS ARE:
- To maintain an open airway.
- To arrange urgent removal to hospital.

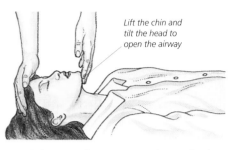

Lift the chin and tilt the head to open the airway

1 If the casualty is unconscious, check breathing and pulse, and place her in the recovery position (*see page 30*).

2 Help a conscious casualty lie down, with the head and shoulders raised and comfortably supported.

IF you suspect spinal injury, treat the casualty as described on pages 156-157.

IF there is discharge from an ear, position the casualty so that the affected ear is lower. Cover the ear with a sterile dressing or clean pad, lightly secured with a bandage. Do not plug the ear.

3 Control any bleeding from the scalp. Look for, and treat, other injuries.

4 Dial 999 for an ambulance. Check and record breathing and pulse rate, and level of response, at 10-minute intervals (*see page 50*), and accompany the casualty to hospital.

CEREBRAL COMPRESSION

This is a very serious condition that almost invariably requires surgery. It occurs when pressure is exerted on the brain within the skull, by, for example, an accumulation of blood or by swelling of an injured brain. It is often associated with head injury and skull fracture, but can be due to other causes (stroke, infection or tumour). It may develop immediately after a head injury, or may be delayed for some hours, or even days.

Compression caused by bleeding

Accumulated blood may clot to press on the brain

RECOGNITION

As compression develops, there will be:
- A deterioration in the level of response.

There may be:
- A recent head injury. The casualty might apparently have made a full recovery but later started to deteriorate, with disorientation and confusion.
- An intense headache.
- Noisy breathing, becoming slow.
- A slow, yet full, strong pulse.
- Unequal pupils.
- Weakness or paralysis on one side of the face or body.
- A raised temperature, and a hot, flushed face.

TREATMENT

Dial 999, and follow the treatment for unconsciousness (*see page 116*).

119

CONVULSIONS

A convulsion, or fit, is a simultaneous, involuntary contraction of many of the body's muscles, caused by a disturbance in the function of the brain. Convulsions are usually accompanied by loss of consciousness.

There are a number of possible causes, including head injury, some brain-damaging diseases, shortage of oxygen to the brain, and the intake of some poisons. In children and infants, fits may be triggered by a high temperature. Fits are also a feature of the condition epilepsy.

No matter what the cause of the fit, you must observe the three rules of treatment for the unconscious casualty (*see page 115*), protect the casualty from further harm during a fit, and arrange appropriate aftercare.

MINOR EPILEPSY

Also known as "petit mal", this is the lesser form of the condition epilepsy, in which brief, sudden disturbances of the brain cause little more than a momentary blurring of consciousness that resembles daydreaming. On recovery, the casualty may simply have lost the thread of what he or she was doing. However, it is not uncommon for a major fit to follow a minor one.

RECOGNITION

There may be:
• Sudden "switching off"; the casualty may be staring blankly ahead.
• Slight twitching movements of lips, eyelids or head.
• Strange "automatic" movements – lip-smacking, chewing, making odd noises, or fiddling with clothing.

TREATMENT

> YOUR AIM IS:
> • To protect the casualty until she is fully recovered.

1 Help the casualty to sit down in a quiet place, and remove any possible sources of harm – for example, hot drinks – from the vicinity.

2 Talk to her calmly and reassuringly. Do not pester her with questions. Stay with her until you are sure she is herself again.

IF she does not recognise and know about her condition, advise her to see her own doctor.

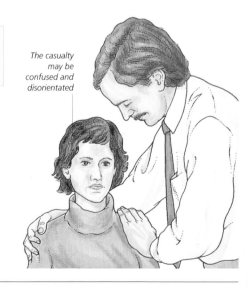

The casualty may be confused and disorientated

MAJOR EPILEPSY

This condition, also known as "grand mal", is characterised by recurrent major disturbances of brain activity, resulting in violent seizures and severe (if temporary) impairment of consciousness. Epileptic fits can be sudden and dramatic, but the casualty may have a brief period of warning – a strange feeling, or special smell or taste – known as an "aura".

RECOGNITION

An epileptic fit usually follows a pattern:
* The casualty suddenly falls unconscious, often letting out a cry.
* He becomes rigid, arching his back (this is known as the *tonic* phase).

* Breathing may cease. The lips may show a blue tinge (*cyanosis*) and the face and neck may become congested.
* Convulsive movements begin (the *clonic* phase). The jaw may be clenched and breathing may be noisy. Saliva may appear at the mouth, blood-stained if lips or tongue have been bitten. There may be loss of bladder or bowel control.
* The muscles relax and breathing becomes normal; the casualty recovers consciousness, usually within a few minutes. He may feel dazed, or behave strangely in a state of "automatism", being unaware of his actions. A fit may also be followed by a deep sleep.

TREATMENT

YOUR AIMS ARE: • To protect the casualty from injury during the fit. • To provide care when consciousness has been regained.

DO NOT lift or move the casualty unless he is in immediate danger. DO NOT use force to restrain him, or put anything in his mouth.

1 If you see the casualty falling, try to support him or ease his fall. Make space around him and ask bystanders to move away.

2 Loosen clothing around his neck and, if possible, protect his head.

3 When the convulsions cease, place him in the recovery position (*see page 30*). Stay with him until he is completely recovered.

IF the casualty is having his first fit, repeated fits, or is unconscious for more than 10 minutes, dial 999 for an ambulance. Note the time and duration of the fit.

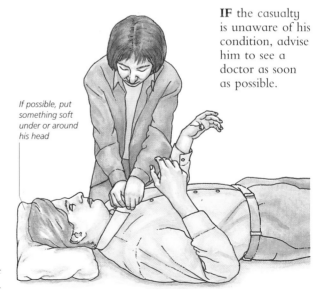

If possible, put something soft under or around his head

IF the casualty is unaware of his condition, advise him to see a doctor as soon as possible.

CONVULSIONS IN YOUNG CHILDREN

Although young children can have epileptic fits just like adults, they may, more commonly, develop convulsions at the onset of an infectious disease or a throat or ear infection associated with a greatly raised body temperature (fever).

These *febrile* convulsions can be alarming, but they are rarely dangerous if properly managed. However, for safety's sake the child should be seen at a hospital to eliminate any serious condition. This may distress the parents further; reassure them that in the vast majority of cases, no further problems will occur once the fit has passed.

RECOGNITION

There will be:
• Clear signs of fever: hot, flushed skin and perhaps sweating.
• Violent muscle twitching, with clenched fists and an arched back.

There may be:
• Twitching of the face with squinting, fixed, or upturned eyes.
• Breath-holding, with congestion of the face and neck.
• Drooling at the mouth.

See also: Unconsciousness, *page 115.*

TREATMENT

Sponging will cool the child

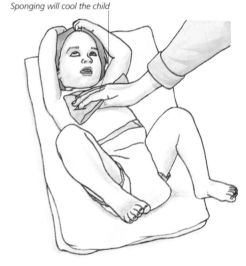

YOUR AIMS ARE:
• To protect the child from injury.
• To cool the child.
• To reassure the parents.
• To arrange removal to hospital.

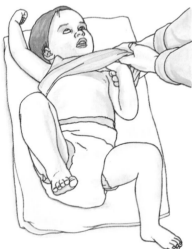

1 Remove any clothes or covering bedclothes. Ensure a good supply of cool, fresh air (though be careful not to overcool the child).

2 Sponge the child with tepid water; start at the head and work down.

3 Position pillows or soft padding so that even violent movement will not result in injury.

4 Keep the airway open, by using the recovery position (*page 30*) if possible.

5 Dial 999 for an ambulance, reassuring the parents.

STROKE

This term is used to describe a condition in which the blood supply to part of the brain is suddenly and seriously impaired, by a blood clot, or a ruptured artery.

Strokes are more common in later life, and in those who suffer from high blood pressure or other circulatory disorder. The effect of a stroke depends on how much, and which part, of the brain is affected. Major strokes can be fatal, but many people make successful recoveries from minor strokes.

RECOGNITION

There may be:

• A sudden, severe headache.
• A confused, emotional mental state that could be mistaken for drunkenness.
• Sudden or progressive loss of consciousness.
• Signs of weakness or paralysis, possibly (but not always) confined to one side of the body, such as: a drooping, dribbling mouth; slurred or impaired speech; loss of power or movement in the limbs; inequality of the pupils; loss of bladder or bowel control.

See also: Unconsciousness, *page 115.*

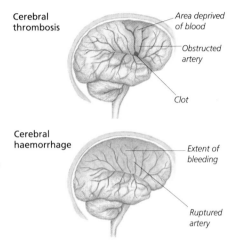

Cerebral thrombosis

Area deprived of blood

Obstructed artery

Clot

Cerebral haemorrhage

Extent of bleeding

Ruptured artery

TREATMENT

YOUR AIMS ARE:
• To maintain an open airway.
• To minimise brain damage.
• To arrange urgent removal to hospital.

1 If the casualty is conscious, lay him down with his head and shoulders slightly raised and supported. Incline his head to one side, and place a towel or cloth so that it will absorb any dribbling.

2 Loosen any constricting clothing that might interfere with breathing.

DO NOT give the casualty anything to eat or drink.

IF the casualty becomes unconscious, check breathing, pulse, and level of response (*see page 115*), and be prepared to resuscitate if necessary. Place him in the recovery position (*see page 30*).

3 Dial 999 for an ambulance.

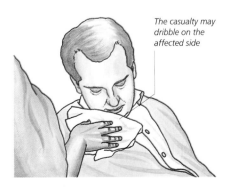

The casualty may dribble on the affected side

OTHER DISORDERS

The nervous system is vulnerable to disorder and damage not only by physical injury and disruptive conditions such as epilepsy, but also by changes in the composition of the blood supplied to the brain.

Chemical changes to which the brain is particularly sensitive include an insufficiency of oxygen in the blood (*see page 54*), altered blood sugar levels, or the presence of toxins such as poisons, alcohol, or drugs.

The problems of substance abuse

The abuse of alcohol, drugs, and other substances is an emotive subject, but you must never let this impair your judgement and management of the unconscious casualty. He or she may be doubly at risk – from not only the dangers of unconsciousness, but also the effects of the intoxicating substance.

The importance of examination

Remember that the symptoms and signs of conditions such as stroke and diabetic emergency can closely resemble, and easily be mistaken for, intoxication. As with any other case of unconsciousness, you should, having ensured an open airway, examine the casualty thoroughly to check for other possible causes.

HYPOGLYCAEMIA

When the blood sugar level falls below normal, the function of the brain is rapidly affected. The condition is known as *hypoglycaemia*, and is most often found in people who suffer from *diabetes mellitus*, commonly known as diabetes (*see opposite*). It can also, more rarely, occur after heavy binge drinking, complicate heat exhaustion and hypothermia, or accompany an epileptic fit.

Emergencies in diabetics

Diabetics are usually aware of their condition, and are well-prepared for emergencies. However, if the "hypo" attack is advanced, consciousness may be impaired or ultimately lost, and your assistance may be vital.

If the casualty is not to his or her knowledge a diabetic, medical advice must be sought, even if the casualty appears to have fully recovered.

Providing that the casualty is conscious, giving sugar can do no harm.

RECOGNITION

There may be:

• A history of diabetes; the casualty recognises the onset of a "hypo" attack.
• Weakness, faintness, or hunger.
• Palpitations and muscle tremors.
• Evidence that the casualty is a diabetic: a warning card or bracelet, sugar lumps, tablets, or an insulin syringe (which may look like a pen) among his possessions.
• Strange actions or behaviour; the casualty may appear confused, belligerent, or even violent.
• Sweating.
• Pallor, and cold, clammy skin.
• A strong, bounding pulse.
• A deteriorating level of response.
• Shallow breathing.

See also: Convulsions, *page 120.*
Heat exhaustion, *page 133.*
Hypothermia, *page 130.*
Unconsciousness, *page 115.*

TREATMENT

> YOUR AIMS ARE:
> • To raise the sugar content of the blood as quickly as possible.
> • To obtain medical aid, urgently if the casualty is unconscious.

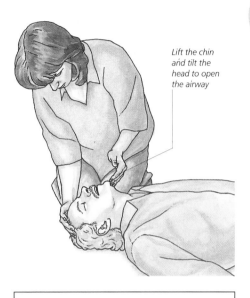

Lift the chin and tilt the head to open the airway

FOR AN UNCONSCIOUS CASUALTY

1 Open the airway, and check and record breathing, pulse, and level of response (*see page 50*). Be prepared to resuscitate if necessary.

2 Turn the casualty into the recovery position (*see page 30*).

3 Dial 999 for an ambulance.

FOR A CONSCIOUS CASUALTY

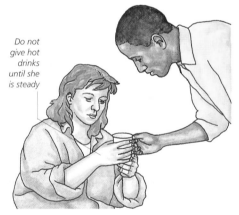

Do not give hot drinks until she is steady

1 Help the casualty to sit or lie down, and give her a sugary drink, sugar lumps, chocolate, or other sweet food.

2 If the casualty's condition improves quickly, give more sweet food or drink, and let her rest until she feels fully recovered. Advise her to see her doctor.

IF her condition does not improve, examine her for other causes of confusion and tremor, and treat as necessary.

Diabetes mellitus

This is a condition in which the body fails to regulate the concentration of sugar (*glucose*) in the blood.

An organ called the pancreas normally produces a hormone, insulin, that controls blood sugar levels. Without insulin, sugar accumulates in the blood, causing *hyperglycaemia*. Diabetics must balance the amount of sugar in their diet with insulin injections or tablets; too much insulin and too little sugar can cause *hypoglycaemia*.

Most diabetics are aware of the risk of hypoglycaemia if, for example, they miss a meal or over-exert themselves, and may carry sugar lumps or glucose tablets to raise their blood sugar level quickly.

Hyperglycaemia
Prolonged high blood sugar can result in unconsciousness, but the diabetic is likely to drift into this state over several days. The signs of this type of diabetic coma are dry skin, a rapid pulse, deep, laboured breathing, and possibly a faint smell of acetone (nail-varnish remover) on the casualty's breath. Urgent hospital treatment is required.

DRUNKENNESS

The unconscious drunkard is at risk from a blocked airway, especially if he or she is lying face-up, or has vomited. There may be head or neck injuries resulting from an assault or fall, or a stroke (see page 123) may have occurred.

Fits are common in binge drinking, and there is also a risk of hypothermia.

See also: Alcohol poisoning, *page 170*.
Hypothermia, *page 130*.
Unconsciousness, *page 115*.

TREATMENT

YOUR AIM IS:
• To maintain an open airway, and obtain medical aid if necessary.

1 Open the casualty's airway, making sure there is no vomit causing obstruction. Check breathing, pulse, and level of response (see page 115), and be prepared to resuscitate if necessary.

2 Quickly but thoroughly, look for, and treat, any associated injuries.

3 Place the casualty in the recovery position (see page 30). Keep a close watch on his or her condition. If in doubt, take or send the casualty to hospital.

IF the casualty is totally unresponsive (for example, to a firm pinch on the hand) or is fitting, dial 999 for an ambulance.

SUBSTANCE ABUSE

A variety of illicit or non-prescribed drugs and substances may deliberately be taken for "kicks", by mouth, by injection, or by inhalation. Some of these can cause unconsciousness and severely impair breathing. If you are in doubt about the cause of unconsciousness, particularly if treating a casualty in unusual circumstances, suspect drug abuse or overdose.

See also: Drug poisoning, *page 168*.
Unconsciousness, *page 115*.

TREATMENT

YOUR AIM IS:
• To maintain an open airway until medical aid is obtained.

1 Open the airway, and check breathing, pulse, and level of response (see page 115). Be prepared to resuscitate if necessary.

2 Place the casualty in the recovery position (see page 30).

3 Dial 999 for an ambulance. Monitor breathing and pulse closely.

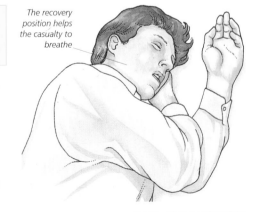
The recovery position helps the casualty to breathe

EFFECTS OF
HEAT AND COLD

The human body is designed to work best at, or close to, a temperature of 37°C (98.6°F). To maintain this temperature, the body possesses mechanisms that generate and conserve heat when the environment is cold, and, conversely, that lose heat when it is hot. These mechanisms are controlled by a special centre in the brain. In addition, man controls his environment to some degree through clothing, heating, and air-conditioning. These make it easier for the body to perform well in a wide range of temperatures. In spite of all this, excessive heat or cold can cause injury and, in extreme cases, serious or even fatal conditions.

The dangers of extreme temperatures

The harmful effects of extreme heat or cold can be localised, as in the case of sunburn, frostbite, or trench foot; or generalised, as with heat exhaustion, heatstroke, and hypothermia. The generalised effects of extremes of temperature tend to be more marked in the very young and the very old, whose temperature-regulation systems may, respectively, be under-developed or impaired.

CONTENTS

THE FIRST AIDER SHOULD:

• Remove, or protect, the casualty from excessively hot or cold surroundings.

• Restore normal body temperature: if the condition was rapid in onset (for example, heatstroke), reverse it rapidly; if it has developed slowly (for example, hypothermia of slow onset affecting an elderly person), the casualty's body temperature must be brought gradually back to normal.

• Obtain appropriate medical attention.

THE BODY TEMPERATURE

To keep the body temperature within a safe range of 36°-38°C (97.8°-100.4°F), the body must maintain a constant balance between heat gain and heat loss. The balance is regulated by a "thermostat" deep within the base of the brain.

The body's steady heat gain, produced by the conversion of food to energy (the *metabolism*) and by muscular activity, must in normal conditions be offset by continuous heat loss. Some methods of heat loss are passive – for example, the natural tendency of body heat to be lost to cool surrounding air. Others are active – notably, changes that occur within the circulatory system and at the skin. In hot conditions, blood vessels dilate in order that more blood heat may be lost by radiation from the skin. This process is reversed when heat must be conserved.

How the body keeps warm

Heat is generated in the tissues by:
• The conversion of food to energy in the body's cells.
• Muscle activity, either voluntary (exercise) or, in cold conditions, involuntary (shivering).

Heat is absorbed:
• From outside sources – the sun, fire, hot air, hot food or drink, or any hot object in contact with the skin.

In cold conditions, the body conserves heat by:
• Constricting blood vessels at the body surface to keep warm blood at the core.
• Reducing sweating.
• Erecting body hairs to "trap" warm air at the skin.

How the body loses heat

Heat may be lost to:
• Cool surrounding air – by radiating from the skin, and in the breath.
• Cool objects in contact with the skin, which provide a "pathway" by which heat escapes.

In hot conditions, the body reacts to lose heat:
• The blood vessels in or near the skin dilate in order to lose blood heat.
• Sweat glands become active. Heat is lost as the sweat evaporates in cooler air.
• The rate and depth of breathing will increase – warm air is expelled, and cool air drawn in to replace it, cooling the blood in the vessels of the lungs.

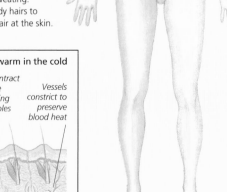

Keeping warm in the cold

Muscles contract to erect the hairs, forming goose pimples

Vessels constrict to preserve blood heat

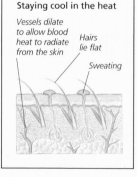

Staying cool in the heat

Vessels dilate to allow blood heat to radiate from the skin

Hairs lie flat

Sweating

THE EFFECTS OF EXTREME COLD

The body reacts to cold by shutting down blood vessels in the skin to prevent "core heat" escaping. Deprived of warm blood, parts such as fingers or toes may, in extreme conditions, actually freeze, causing injury (*frostbite*). If the core temperature becomes dangerously low, bodily functions slow down (the condition known as *hypothermia*) and may stop altogether.

FROSTBITE

This typically occurs in freezing and often dry and windy conditions. Casualties who cannot move are particularly vulnerable. The tissues of the extremities freeze, causing damage which may be superficial or deep; minor cases ("frostnip") recover well, but severe frostbite can result in permanent damage.

RECOGNITION

There may be:
- At first, "pins-and-needles"; the affected part becomes pale.
- The part becomes numb. Its skin may feel hard and stiff, turning white, then mottled and blue, and eventually black.

TREATMENT

YOUR AIMS ARE:
- To warm the affected area slowly, to prevent further tissue damage.
- To obtain medical aid if necessary.

IF a long walk or further exposure to intense cold is unavoidable, do not thaw the part until shelter is reached.

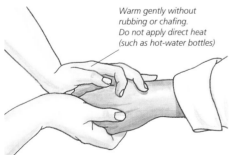

Warm gently without rubbing or chafing. Do not apply direct heat (such as hot-water bottles)

1 Very gently remove any gloves, rings, or boots. Warm the part gently with your hands or in your lap, or in the casualty's armpit.

2 Get the casualty to warm surroundings; if the feet are affected, carry him if possible.

3 If colour does not return rapidly to the skin, place the affected part in warm water. Dry it very carefully, and apply a light dressing of fluffed dry gauze, bandaged *without pressure*. Do not burst any blisters.

4 Raise and support the limb to reduce swelling. The casualty may take two paracetamol tablets to relieve pain. If necessary, take or send him to hospital.

Immersion (Trench) foot
This may be caused by prolonged exposure to near-freezing temperatures in damp, slushy conditions. Lack of mobility, tight boots and wet socks all increase the risk.

In the early stages the feet are white, cold, and numb; later they become red, hot, and very painful, and blisters may form. Treatment is as for frostbite.

129

HYPOTHERMIA

This condition develops when the body temperature falls below 35°C (95°F). The effects vary with the speed of onset, and the level to which the temperature falls.

Degrees of severity

Moderate hypothermia can usually be completely reversed. Deep hypothermia (core temperature below 26°C/79°F) is often, though not always, fatal: it is *always* worthwhile persisting with resuscitation until a doctor decides otherwise.

How hypothermia can be caused

"Accidental hypothermia" *(see page 132)* is caused by prolonged exposure to cold outdoors, especially in wet and windy conditions. Moving air has a much greater cooling effect than still air; the "wind-chill factor" can, therefore, substantially increase the risk.

Death from cold water immersion may be caused by hypothermia rather than drowning. When the body is surrounded by cold water, cooling is 30 times faster than in dry air, and a dangerously low body temperature can be reached within a relatively short time.

Hypothermia in the home

This condition may develop over several days in poorly-heated houses. Infants, and frail, thin, and elderly people, are particularly vulnerable. Lack of agility, chronic illness, fatigue, hunger, and dehydration all increase the risk.

RECOGNITION

As hypothermia develops, there may be:
• Shivering.
• Cold, pale, dry skin; the body feels "as cold as marble".
• Apathy, confusion, or irrational behaviour; occasionally belligerence.
• Lethargy.
• Failing consciousness.
• Slow and shallow breathing.
• A slow and weakening pulse.
• In extreme cases, cardiac arrest.

Hypothermia in the elderly

Frail, infirm, and elderly people are at risk from hypothermia if the weather is very cold. They often go without adequate food or heating, and may also be relatively immobile.

Treating the elderly

Hypothermia in the home may often develop slowly, and rewarming should also be gradual. Rapid warming (for example, in a hot bath) may send cold blood from the body surfaces to the heart and brain too suddenly. Always call a doctor, because these cases may disguise the symptoms of, or accompany, a stroke or heart attack.

Preventing hypothermia in the home

Ensure rooms are heated sufficiently. Wear several layers of warm clothing, and take adequate hot meals and drinks.

Hypothermia in infants

A baby's temperature-regulating mechanisms are under-developed, and hypothermia may develop in a cold room.

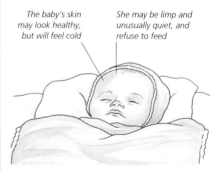

The baby's skin may look healthy, but will feel cold

She may be limp and unusually quiet, and refuse to feed

Rewarm a hypothermic baby gradually. Wrap her in blankets and warm the room. A doctor *must* examine the child.

FOR A CASUALTY AT HOME OR IN SHELTER

An otherwise fit casualty who has become chilled outdoors may be warmed by bathing

YOUR AIMS ARE:
- To prevent the casualty losing more body heat.
- To rewarm the casualty.

IF you have brought the casualty indoors then, providing she is fit and able to climb into the bath unaided, she may be rewarmed quickly in a hot bath (40°C/ 104° F). Otherwise, quickly remove her coat and shoes, and replace any wet clothing with warm, dry garments.

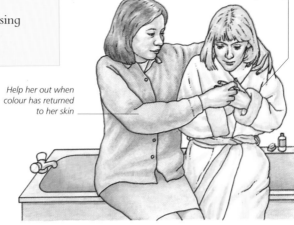

Help her out when colour has returned to her skin

1 Put the casualty in bed, well-covered.

A frail or elderly casualty should be allowed to warm up gradually in bed

Cover the casualty's head for additional warmth

DO NOT place heat sources, such as hot-water bottles, next to the casualty. These speed up blood flow through the skin, and may cause an "after-drop" in the core temperature as cold blood returns from the body surfaces.

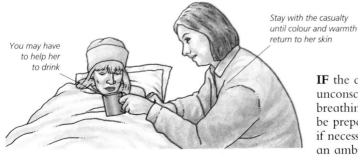

You may have to help her to drink

Stay with the casualty until colour and warmth return to her skin

2 Give a conscious casualty hot drinks, soup, or high-energy foods such as chocolate.

3 If in doubt about the casualty's condition, or if the casualty is elderly or an infant, call a doctor.

IF the casualty becomes unconscious, check breathing and pulse, and be prepared to resuscitate if necessary. Dial 999 for an ambulance. You *must* continue resuscitation, if it is necessary, while the casualty re-warms until medical help arrives.

FOR A CASUALTY IN THE OPEN

YOUR AIMS ARE:
- To prevent the casualty losing more body heat.
- To rewarm the casualty.

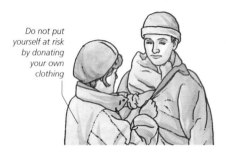

Do not put yourself at risk by donating your own clothing

1 Insulate the casualty with extra clothing, waterproofs, or blankets, remembering to cover his head.

2 Take or carry the casualty to a sheltered place as quickly as possible.

Preventing accidental hypothermia

Outdoor expeditions must be carefully planned, and participants should be properly trained. Those with even minor illness on the day should not take part, and anyone who becomes unwell or is injured during the expedition should be taken to a place of safety without delay.

Be equipped for an emergency
Always take a spare sweater, dry socks, dry and well-aired sleeping bags, and a survival bag. Take extra high-energy food and drink, but not alcohol; it dilates the blood vessels, and thus accelerates heat loss.

Dress to beat the cold
Layers of clothing are more effective than one warm garment. The outer layer should be wind- and waterproof, and able to be loosened at the neck and wrists.
  If you fall into cold water you should, in order to reduce heat loss, keep all your clothes on except very heavy coats and boots, which may drag you down.

Shelter and warm him with your body

A polythene survival bag will protect him from wind and rain

IF the casualty becomes unconscious, check breathing and pulse, and be prepared to resuscitate if necessary. You *must*, until help arrives, continue resuscitation while the casualty re-warms.

Lay the casualty on a thick layer of dry insulating material, such as heather or bracken

3 Protect the casualty from the ground and the elements – put him in a dry sleeping bag, cover him with blankets or newspapers, or enclose him in a polythene survival bag.

4 Send for help. Ideally, two people should go, provided there is someone to remain with the casualty.

5 Providing the casualty is conscious, give him hot drinks if available.

6 When help arrives, evacuate the casualty to hospital by stretcher.

THE EFFECTS OF EXTREME HEAT

In extremely hot conditions, the body's heat-loss mechanisms (*see page 128*) may fail. When the atmospheric temperature equals the body temperature, it becomes impossible for the body to lose heat by radiation. If there is also high humidity (when the air is laden with moisture), sweat does not evaporate well. In these circumstances, particularly during strenuous exercise when extra heat is generated by muscular activity, heat exhaustion, or the more dangerous condition, heatstroke, may develop.

HEAT EXHAUSTION

This condition usually develops gradually, and is caused by loss of salt and water from the body through excessive sweating. It is more common in persons who are unaccustomed to working or exercising in a hot, humid environment, and in those who are unwell, especially with diarrhoea and vomiting.

RECOGNITION

As the condition develops, there may be:
- Headache, dizziness, and confusion.
- Loss of appetite, and nausea.
- Sweating, with pale, clammy skin.
- Cramps in the limbs or abdomen.
- Rapid, weakening pulse and breathing.

TREATMENT

YOUR AIMS ARE:
- To move the casualty to cool surroundings.
- To replace lost fluid and salt.

1 Help the casualty to lie down in a cool place. Raise and support her legs.

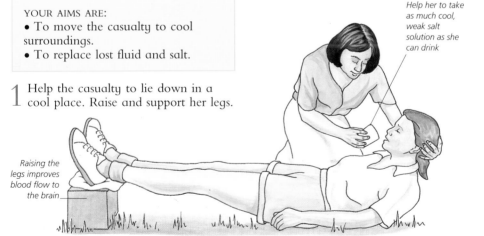

Help her to take as much cool, weak salt solution as she can drink

Raising the legs improves blood flow to the brain

2 Provided she is conscious, help her to sip plenty of weak salt solution (one teaspoon per litre of water).

3 If recovery is rapid, advise the casualty to see her own doctor.

IF the casualty becomes unconscious, place her in the recovery position (*see page 30*). Dial 999 for an ambulance. Check and record breathing, pulse, and level of response (*see page 50*) every 10 minutes.

HEATSTROKE

This condition often occurs suddenly, and can cause unconsciousness in minutes. There may be a warning period when the casualty feels uneasy and unwell.

Heatstroke is caused by a failure of the "thermostat" in the brain, due either to prolonged exposure to very hot surroundings, or illness involving a very high fever (such as malaria). The body rapidly becomes dangerously overheated.

RECOGNITION

There may be:
- Headache, dizziness, and discomfort.
- Restlessness and confusion.
- Hot, flushed, and dry skin.
- A rapid deterioration in the level of response (*see page 115*).
- A full, bounding pulse.
- Body temperature above 40°C (104°F).

TREATMENT

> YOUR AIMS ARE:
> - To lower the casualty's body temperature as quickly as possible.
> - To obtain medical attention.

1 Move the casualty quickly to a cool place. Remove all outer clothing. Call a doctor.

IF the casualty becomes unconscious, lay her down, check breathing and pulse, and be prepared to resuscitate if necessary. Dial 999 for an ambulance. Place the casualty in the recovery position (*see page 30*).

Keep the sheet wet by continually sprinkling it with water

Fan the casualty to keep her cool

2 Wrap the casualty in a cold, wet sheet, and keep it wet. Cool her until the under-the-tongue temperature falls to 38°C (100.4°F).

3 When the temperature has fallen to a safe level (38°C/100.4°F), replace the wet sheet with a dry one. Continue to observe the casualty carefully.

IF the temperature rises again, repeat the cooling process (step 2).

134

BONE, JOINT, AND MUSCLE INJURIES

The skeleton is the framework around which the body is built, and on which all the tissues of the body depend for support. In order that we may move, the skeleton is jointed in many places. Muscles attached to the bones work to make them move. These movements are controlled by the will, and co-ordinated by specialised nerves.

What you will find in this chapter

The first section of this chapter looks at how the musculoskeletal system works, and how and why it can be injured. General treatment principles for the various types of injury are laid out. Following that, specific first aid treatments for injuries to bones, joints, and muscles in every part of the body, from top to toe, are given.

The only type of fracture not covered in these pages is skull fracture, which, because of its potential effect on the brain, is discussed in the chapter *Disorders of Consciousness (pages 113–126)*.

THE FIRST AIDER SHOULD:

• Steady and support the injured part with your hands.

• Find more permanent support for the injured part. Soft tissue injuries will benefit from padding and firm bandaging, while fractures and dislocations may need splinting. An uninjured part of the casualty's body provides a natural form of support.

• If a broken bone lies within a large bulk of tissue (for example, the thigh), treat the casualty for shock.

• Obtain medical attention. Hospital treatment will be required for all but the most minor injuries.

CONTENTS

BONES, JOINTS, AND MUSCLES

The body is built on a framework of bones – the skeleton – that supports the muscles, blood vessels and nerves of the body, and gives protection to certain organs. Movement is made possible by muscles attached to the bones, and by movable joints where bones meet.

THE SKELETON

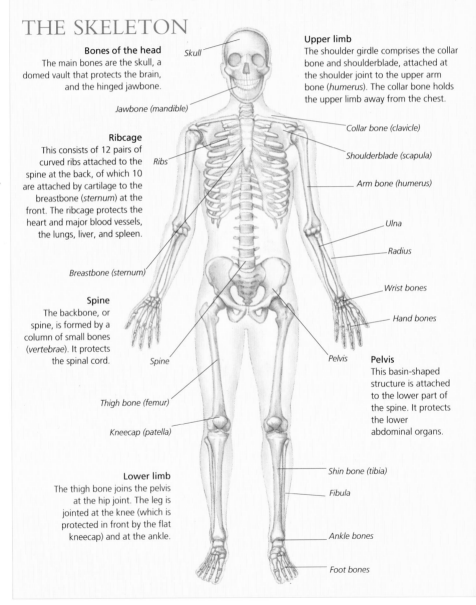

Bones of the head
The main bones are the skull, a domed vault that protects the brain, and the hinged jawbone.

Skull

Jawbone (mandible)

Ribcage
This consists of 12 pairs of curved ribs attached to the spine at the back, of which 10 are attached by cartilage to the breastbone (*sternum*) at the front. The ribcage protects the heart and major blood vessels, the lungs, liver, and spleen.

Ribs

Breastbone (sternum)

Spine
The backbone, or spine, is formed by a column of small bones (*vertebrae*). It protects the spinal cord.

Spine

Thigh bone (femur)

Kneecap (patella)

Lower limb
The thigh bone joins the pelvis at the hip joint. The leg is jointed at the knee (which is protected in front by the flat kneecap) and at the ankle.

Upper limb
The shoulder girdle comprises the collar bone and shoulderblade, attached at the shoulder joint to the upper arm bone (*humerus*). The collar bone holds the upper limb away from the chest.

Collar bone (clavicle)

Shoulderblade (scapula)

Arm bone (humerus)

Ulna

Radius

Wrist bones

Hand bones

Pelvis

Pelvis
This basin-shaped structure is attached to the lower part of the spine. It protects the lower abdominal organs.

Shin bone (tibia)

Fibula

Ankle bones

Foot bones

THE JOINTS

Wherever one bone meets another, there is a joint. Joints are of two main types: movable and immovable.

Movable joints allow movement between adjacent bones and are of three types: slightly movable, ball-and-socket, and hinge joints (*see below*).

Immovable joints are those where the bone edges fit firmly into each other, or where the bones are fused together (for example, the skull), so that no movement can take place.

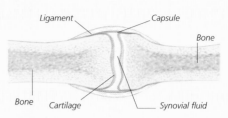

Structure of a movable joint
Bone ends are covered in smooth cartilage that minimises friction. Bands of strong, fibrous tissue (*ligaments*) bind the bone ends together. The joint is enclosed in a capsule filled with a lubricant (the *synovial fluid*).

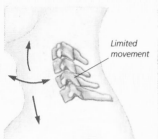

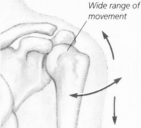

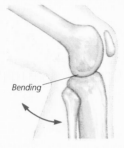

Slightly movable joints
These are shaped to allow only slight gliding or rocking movements. Examples are the joints between the vertebrae, and those between the ribs and spine.

Ball-and-socket joints
The round head of one bone fits into the cup-shaped cavity of another. The swivelling action allows movement in all directions. Examples are the shoulder and hip.

Hinge joints
The surfaces of the bone ends are contoured together to allow bending (*flexion*) and straightening (*extension*) in only one plane. Examples are the elbow and knee.

THE MUSCLES

Muscles cause the various parts of the body to move by the contraction and relaxation of their fibres.

Voluntary muscles are so-called because they are controlled by the will. These muscles are attached to the bones by bands of strong, fibrous tissue (*tendons*). They operate in groups: as one group of muscles contracts, its paired group relaxes.

Involuntary muscles operate the internal organs and work continuously, even when we are asleep. They are controlled by the autonomic nervous system (*see page 114*).

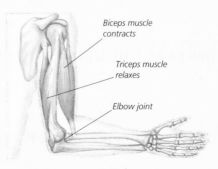

How voluntary muscles work together in the arm
The *biceps* contracts to become shorter, drawing the lower arm towards it. Its opposite muscle, the *triceps*, relaxes to allow the arm to bend at the elbow.

137

TYPES OF INJURY

Bones may be broken (*fractured*), displaced at a joint (*dislocated*), or both. Dislocation is usually caused by a wrenching force, and often tears the joint's ligaments. Muscles, and the tendons which attach them to bones, may also be strained or torn. It can be difficult for the First Aider to distinguish between the various types of *musculoskeletal* injury.

FRACTURES

A fracture is a break or crack in a bone. Bones are not brittle structures like blackboard chalk, but tough and resilient. Bones behave like the branches of a healthy tree when struck or twisted. Generally, considerable force is required to break a bone, but old or diseased bones become brittle and can easily break or crumble under stress.

Conversely, young bones that are still growing are supple and may split, bend, or crack just like a young sapling – hence the name "greenstick fracture" for this type of injury.

Any type of fracture may be associated with an open wound, and complicated by injury to adjoining muscles, blood vessels, nerves, and organs.

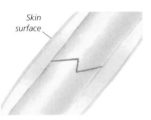

Skin surface

Simple fracture
This is, simply, a clean break or crack in a bone.

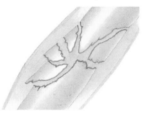

Comminuted fracture
This term is applied to a fracture with multiple bone fragments.

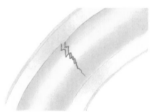

Greenstick fracture
A split in a young, immature bone, common in children.

How fractures are caused

Fractures caused by direct force
A bone may break at a point where a heavy blow is received. For example, the shin bone may be broken by the impact of a moving vehicle's bumper.

Fractures caused by indirect force
Force may travel from the point of impact through the body to break bones elsewhere. Indirect force may also be produced by a twist or wrench: a trip or stumble can break a leg bone, for example. Rarely, violent muscle contraction fractures a bone to which the muscle is attached.

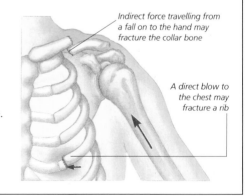

Indirect force travelling from a fall on to the hand may fracture the collar bone

A direct blow to the chest may fracture a rib

OPEN AND CLOSED FRACTURES

Open, or compound, fractures are accompanied by a wound; the overlying skin is broken and the bone may be exposed to contamination from the skin surface and the air.

When the skin around a broken bone is intact, the injury is known as a closed fracture. There will often be bruising and swelling.

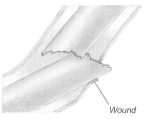

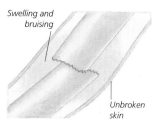

Swelling and bruising

Wound

Unbroken skin

Open fracture
The wound may be caused by the injuring force, or from within by bone fragments perforating the skin.

Closed fracture
The surrounding skin is unbroken; internal injury to surrounding tissues may cause local swelling.

DISLOCATIONS

Displacement of a bone at a joint (*dislocation*) can be caused by a strong force wrenching the bone into an abnormal position, or by violent muscle contraction. There may be associated tearing of the ligaments (*see below*). The joints most often dislocated are the shoulder, thumb, finger and jaw. It can often be difficult to distinguish a dislocation from a fracture.

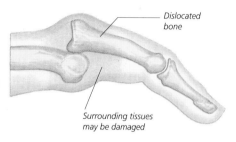

Dislocated bone

Surrounding tissues may be damaged

SOFT TISSUE INJURIES

These are injuries that affect the ligaments and the muscles. A *sprain* is an injury to a ligament at, or near, a joint, and is most frequently caused by a wrenching movement at the joint that tears the surrounding tissues.

Muscles and their tendons may be overstretched and torn by violent or sudden movement. Muscle damage can occur in one of three ways:
• *Strain* A partial tearing of the muscle, often at the junction of the muscle and the tendon that joins it to a bone.
• *Rupture* Complete tearing of the muscle, which may occur in the fleshy part or in the tendon.
• *Deep bruising* This may be extensive where there is a large bulk of muscle.

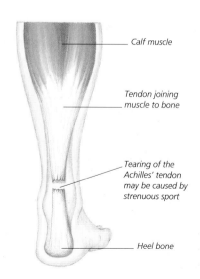

Calf muscle

Tendon joining muscle to bone

Tearing of the Achilles' tendon may be caused by strenuous sport

Heel bone

ASSESSMENT OF BONE, JOINT, AND MUSCLE INJURIES

Some injuries are obvious, such as an open fracture, or a dislocated thumb. Others may only be revealed by X-ray examination. When you are assessing an injury, note as many features as possible, without any unnecessary movement of the injured part. Try to visualise how the

injury was caused, and how much force might have been involved. Compare the shape, position, and appearance of the injured part with the same area on the uninjured side. If you are in doubt about the severity of an injury, you should always treat it as a fracture.

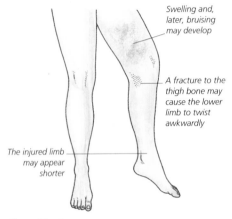

Swelling and, later, bruising may develop

A fracture to the thigh bone may cause the lower limb to twist awkwardly

The injured limb may appear shorter

Signs of fracture
You may notice a shortening, bending, or twisting of the limb. Coarse grating of the bone ends (*crepitus*) may be heard or felt (*do not* try to produce this deliberately). Swelling and bruising may develop at the fracture site.

RECOGNITION

There may have been:
• A recent violent blow, or a fall.
• The snapping sound of a broken bone or torn ligament.
• The sharp pain of a muscle tear.

There may be:
• Difficulty in moving a limb normally, or at all (for example, inability to walk).
• Pain at or near the site of injury, made worse by movement. Severe and "sickening" pain often indicates dislocation; tenderness over a bone if gently touched is a sign of fracture.
• Distortion, swelling, and bruising.
• Signs of shock, if the fracture is to the thigh bone, ribcage, or pelvis.

See also: Shock, *page 68*.

Stable and unstable injuries

Stable injuries
The force causing what is known as a "stable injury" may either fail to break the bone completely, or may act in such a way that the broken ends are impacted, or jammed together. Such injuries are fairly common at the wrist, shoulder, ankle, and hip. Because there is little movement at the site, stable injuries can usually be gently handled without causing more damage.

Unstable injuries
With this type of injury, the bone is completely broken, or the ligaments are ruptured, in such a way that a broken bone or bone end may be displaced. Such injuries require very careful handling in order to avoid causing further internal damage.

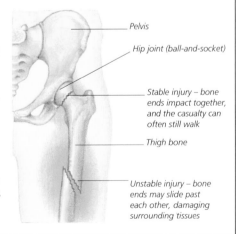

Pelvis

Hip joint (ball-and-socket)

Stable injury – bone ends impact together, and the casualty can often still walk

Thigh bone

Unstable injury – bone ends may slide past each other, damaging surrounding tissues

TREATMENT FOR CLOSED FRACTURES AND DISLOCATIONS

YOUR AIMS ARE:
- To prevent movement at the site of injury.
- To arrange removal to hospital, maintaining comfortable support during transport.

DO NOT move the casualty until the injured part is secured and supported, unless he is in danger.

DO NOT let the casualty have anything to eat or drink.

Traction
If a fractured limb is bent or angled so that you cannot immobilise it, you may apply traction to gently pull it straight. This overcomes the pull of the muscles, and reduces pain and bleeding at the fracture site.

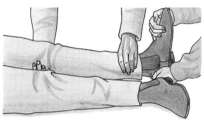

Applying traction
Pull steadily in the line of the bone until the limb is securely immobilised. You can do no harm provided that you pull only in a straight line, but *do not* persist if traction causes intolerable pain.

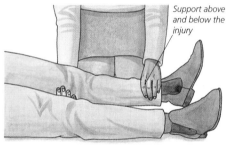

Support above and below the injury

1 Tell the casualty to keep still, and steady and support the injured part with your hands until it is immobilised.

Tie knots on the uninjured side

Immobilise joints above and below a fracture site

Insert soft padding between bony points, and to fill hollows

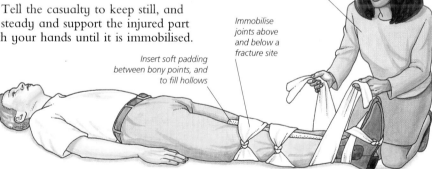

2 For firmer support, secure the injured part to a sound part of the body.
- *For upper limb fractures,* always support the arm against the trunk with a sling and, if necessary, bandaging.
- *For lower limb fractures,* if removal to hospital will be delayed, bandage the sound leg to the injured one (*as above*).

IF you suspect dislocation, do not try to replace the bone in its socket.

3 Dial 999 for an ambulance. Treat the casualty for shock, if necessary (*see page 68*). If possible, raise the injured limb. Check the circulation (*see page 205*) beyond any bandages every 10 minutes.

TREATMENT FOR OPEN FRACTURES

YOUR AIMS ARE:
• To prevent blood loss, movement and infection at the site of injury.
• To arrange removal to hospital, maintaining comfortable support during transport.

DO NOT move the casualty until the injured part is secured and supported, unless she is in danger.

DO NOT let the casualty have anything to eat or drink.

1 If you can, get help to support the limb while you work on the wound.

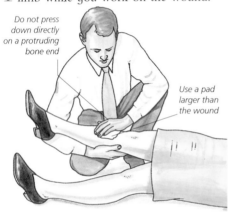

Do not press down directly on a protruding bone end

Use a pad larger than the wound

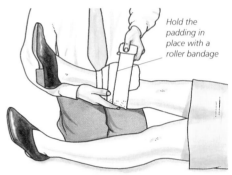

Hold the padding in place with a roller bandage

IF bone is protruding, build up pads of soft, non-fluffy material around the bone until you can bandage over the pads.

2 Cover the wound with a sterile dressing or clean pad, and apply pressure to control bleeding (*see page 78*).

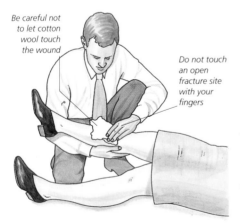

Be careful not to let cotton wool touch the wound

Do not touch an open fracture site with your fingers

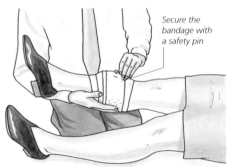

Secure the bandage with a safety pin

4 Secure the dressing and padding; bandage firmly, but not so tightly that the circulation is impeded.

5 Immobilise as for a closed fracture (*see page 141*), keeping the injured part elevated if possible.

6 Dial 999 for an ambulance, and treat the casualty for shock (*see page 68*). Check the circulation beyond the bandaging (*see page 205*) every 10 minutes.

3 Place cotton wool or padding over and around the dressing.

TREATMENT FOR SOFT TISSUE INJURIES

Sprains, strains and deep bruising are all initially treated by following the "RICE" procedure (*see right*). This treatment may suffice, but if you are in doubt as to the severity of the injury, treat as a fracture (*see page 141*).

> THE **RICE** PROCEDURE:
> **R** Rest the injured part.
> **I** Apply Ice or a cold compress.
> **C** Compress the injury.
> **E** Elevate the injured part.

> YOUR AIMS ARE:
> • To reduce swelling and pain.
> • To obtain medical attention if necessary.

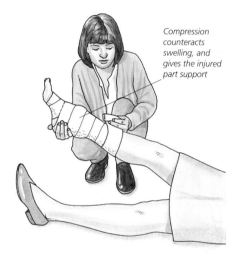

Compression counteracts swelling, and gives the injured part support

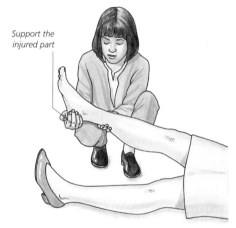

Support the injured part

1 Rest, steady, and support the injured part in the most comfortable position for the casualty.

3 Apply gentle, even pressure to the injured part by surrounding the area with a thick layer of cotton wool or plastic foam, secured with a bandage.

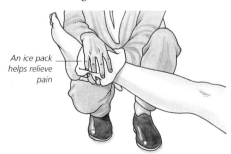

An ice pack helps relieve pain

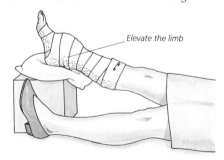

Elevate the limb

2 If the injury happened recently, cool the area by applying an ice pack or cold compress (*see page 203*). This will reduce swelling, bruising, and pain.

4 Raise and support the injured limb, to reduce blood flow to the injury and minimise bruising.

5 Take or send the casualty to hospital or, if the injury seems very minor, advise the casualty to rest the injured part and to see her doctor if necessary.

INJURIES TO THE FACE AND JAW

Common injuries to the face include a broken nose, cheekbone, or jaw. The jaw can also be dislocated. The main danger is obstruction of the airway, either by swollen, displaced, or lacerated tissue, by loose teeth, or by blood and saliva (because the casualty cannot swallow adequately). There may be damage to the brain, skull, or neck.

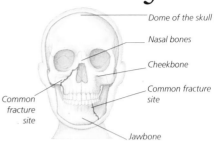

Dome of the skull

Nasal bones

Cheekbone

Common fracture site

Common fracture site

Jawbone

MAJOR FACIAL FRACTURES

These injuries may appear horrifying, with distortion of the eye sockets, nose, upper teeth, and palate. Swelling and bruising may develop rapidly, and there may be bleeding from the nose or mouth.

The danger is that swelling, bleeding, or displaced tissue may block the airway. Check also for head and neck injury.

See also: Head injuries, *page 117.*

TREATMENT

> YOUR AIM IS:
> • To keep the airway open, and arrange urgent removal to hospital.

1 Open and, if necessary, clear the airway.

2 Place the casualty in the recovery position (*see page 30*).

3 Dial 999 for an ambulance.

Transporting the casualty
If you have to carry the casualty on a stretcher, place him or her in the recovery position to protect the airway; or, providing there are no other injuries, lie the casualty face-down on the stretcher, with his or her head beyond the canvas, with the forehead supported by a strap or bandage tied between the handles.

IF the jawbone is injured, place soft padding under the head to keep the weight off the jaw. Do not apply a jaw bandage.

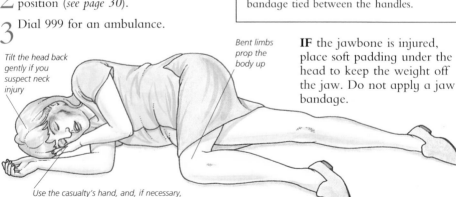

Tilt the head back gently if you suspect neck injury

Bent limbs prop the body up

Use the casualty's hand, and, if necessary, soft padding to support the head

CHEEKBONE AND NOSE FRACTURES

Fractures of the cheekbone and nose are common, and are usually the result of fighting. The associated swelling is uncomfortable, and may block the air passages in the nose. These injuries should always be checked at hospital.

TREATMENT

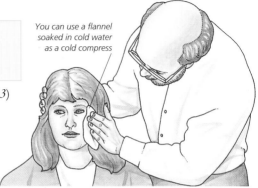

YOUR AIMS ARE:
- To minimise pain and swelling.
- To arrange removal to hospital.

You can use a flannel soaked in cold water as a cold compress

1 Apply a cold compress (*see page 203*) to reduce swelling.

2 Treat an associated nosebleed if necessary (*see page 85*).

3 Take or send the casualty to hospital.

INJURIES TO THE LOWER JAW

Jaw fractures are usually the result of direct force, such as a heavy blow to the jaw. However, a blow to one side of the jaw can sometimes cause a fracture on the other side. A fall on to the point of the chin can fracture both sides. A blow may also dislocate the jaw, as can yawning; dislocation is usually obvious.

RECOGNITION

There may be:
- Pain, often sickening, increased by jaw movement and swallowing.
- Distortion of the teeth, and dribbling.
- Swelling, tenderness, and bruising.
- A wound or bruising inside the mouth.

TREATMENT

YOUR AIM IS:
- To protect the airway while arranging removal to hospital.

IF the casualty is seriously injured, treat as for a major fracture of the face (*see opposite*).

1 For a conscious casualty who is not seriously injured: help her to sit up with her head well forward, to allow any blood, mucus, and saliva to drain away.

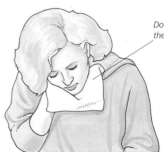

Do not bandage the pad in place

IF she vomits, support her jaw and head, and gently clean out her mouth.

2 Ask the casualty to hold a soft pad firmly in place to support the jaw.

3 Take or send the casualty to hospital, keeping her jaw supported.

145

INJURIES TO THE UPPER LIMB

The term "upper limb" is used to describe the shoulder girdle and the arm. Casualties with injuries to the collar bone, shoulder, and arm can often be transported to hospital as sitting or walking cases.

FRACTURED COLLAR BONE

The two collar bones (*clavicles*) form struts between the breastbone and the shoulderblades, giving support to the arms. They are commonly broken by indirect force, transmitted from a fall on to the out-stretched hand or impact at the shoulder. Fractures of the collar bone caused by a direct blow are rare.

RECOGNITION

There may be:

• Pain and tenderness at the site of the injury, increased by movement.
• Attempts to relax muscles and relieve pain; the casualty may support the arm at the elbow, and incline the head to the injured side.

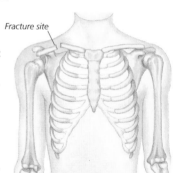

Fracture site

TREATMENT

> YOUR AIMS ARE:
> • To immobilise the upper limb on the injured side.
> • To arrange removal to hospital.

2 Support the arm in an elevation sling (*see page 215*).

3 Secure the arm to her chest with a broad-fold bandage over the sling.

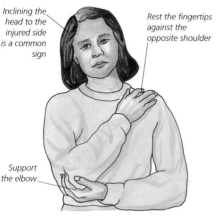

Inclining the head to the injured side is a common sign

Rest the fingertips against the opposite shoulder

Support the elbow

1 Sit the casualty down. Place the arm on her injured side across her chest.

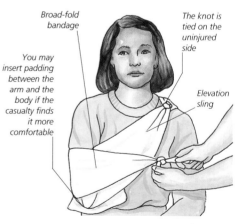

Broad-fold bandage

You may insert padding between the arm and the body if the casualty finds it more comfortable

The knot is tied on the uninjured side

Elevation sling

4 Take or send the casualty to hospital, transporting as a sitting case.

DISLOCATED SHOULDER

A fall on to the shoulder or a wrenching force may cause the head of the arm bone (*humerus*) to come out of the shoulder joint socket. This dislocation is extremely painful, making any movement of the shoulder intolerable. Some people suffer repeated dislocations until a strengthening operation can be carried out.

RECOGNITION

There will be:
- Pain, increased by movement.
- Reluctance to move because of the pain; the casualty often supports the arm, and inclines the head to the injured side.
- A flat, angular appearance to the shoulder.

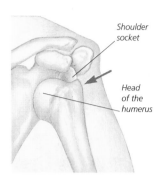

Shoulder socket

Head of the humerus

TREATMENT

> YOUR AIMS ARE:
> - To support the injured limb.
> - To arrange removal to hospital.

1 Sit the casualty down. Gently place the affected arm across her chest at an angle that causes the least pain.

2 Support the limb in an arm sling (*see page 214*).

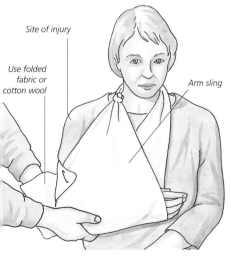

Site of injury

Use folded fabric or cotton wool

Arm sling

3 Insert soft padding between the arm and the chest on the affected side.

Shoulder sprain

A fall on to the point of the shoulder may sprain the ligaments bracing the collar bone at the shoulder. Other sprains, common in older people, affect the capsule and tendons around the shoulder joint. Treat shoulder sprains as for a fractured collar bone (*see opposite*).

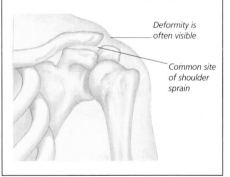

Deformity is often visible

Common site of shoulder sprain

DO NOT attempt to replace the bone in its socket.

DO NOT give the casualty anything to eat or drink, as an anaesthetic may be necessary.

4 Take or send the casualty to hospital, transporting in the sitting position.

FRACTURED UPPER ARM

The long bone of the upper arm may be fractured across its shaft by a direct blow, but it is much more common, especially in the elderly, for the neck of the humerus at the shoulder to break, usually following a fall. Because this is a stable injury (*see page 140*), casualties may put up with the pain and walk around for some time with the fracture unprotected and without seeking medical advice.

RECOGNITION

There will be:
• Pain, increased by movement.

There may be:
• Tenderness over the fracture site.
• Rapid swelling.
• Bruising, which may develop more slowly.

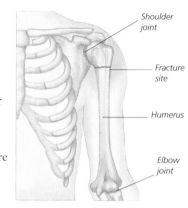

Shoulder joint

Fracture site

Humerus

Elbow joint

TREATMENT

YOUR AIMS ARE:
• To immobilise the arm.
• To arrange removal to hospital.

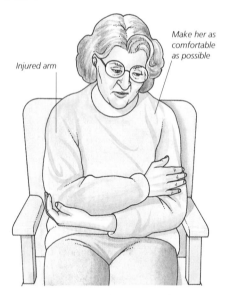

Injured arm

Make her as comfortable as possible

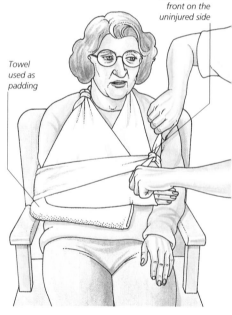

Tie the knot in front on the uninjured side

Towel used as padding

1 Sit the casualty down. Gently place the injured arm across her chest in the position that is most comfortable. Ask her to support her arm, if possible.

2 Support the arm in an arm sling (*see page 214*), and secure the limb to her chest; place soft padding between the arm and chest, and tie a broad-fold bandage around the chest over the sling.

3 Take or send the casualty to hospital, transporting in the sitting position.

INJURIES AROUND THE ELBOW

Fractures at the elbow joint are fairly common, often resulting from a fall on to the hand. A fracture to the head of the radius is characterised by a stiff elbow that cannot be fully straightened.

In children, fracture of the humerus just above the elbow is fairly common. This is an unstable injury; the broken bone ends may move and damage surrounding blood vessels and nerves. It is important to make frequent checks on the circulation at the wrist pulse.

RECOGNITION

There will be:
• Pain, increased by movement.
• Tenderness over the fracture site.
• Possible swelling and bruising.
• If the head of the radius is fractured, a stiff elbow.

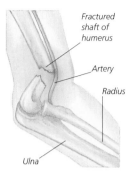

Fractured shaft of humerus

Artery

Radius

Ulna

TREATMENT

> YOUR AIM IS:
> • To immobilise the arm without further injury to the joint.
> • To arrange removal to hospital.

For an injured elbow that can be bent

Treat as for a fracture of the upper arm (*see opposite*). Check for the pulse at the affected wrist every 10 minutes. If it is not present, gently straighten the elbow until the pulse returns and support it in that position.

FOR AN ELBOW THAT CANNOT BE BENT

1 Lay the casualty down, and place the injured limb on his trunk.

> DO NOT attempt to forcibly bend or straighten the elbow.

2 Insert soft padding between the injured limb and his body to ensure that bandaging will not displace the broken bones.

3 Bandage the injured limb to the trunk, first at the wrist and hips, then above and below the elbow.

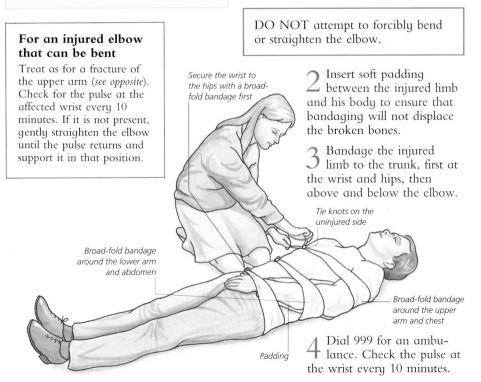

Secure the wrist to the hips with a broad-fold bandage first

Tie knots on the uninjured side

Broad-fold bandage around the lower arm and abdomen

Broad-fold bandage around the upper arm and chest

Padding

4 Dial 999 for an ambulance. Check the pulse at the wrist every 10 minutes.

149

INJURIES TO THE FOREARM AND WRIST

The bones of the forearm (the *radius* and *ulna*) may be fractured across their shafts by a heavy blow. Because the bones have little fleshy covering, these fractures are often open – associated with a wound.

The most common fracture around the wrist is a Colles' fracture (*see right*), usually sustained by older women who fall on to an outstretched hand. In a young adult this may break one of the small bones in the wrist. The complex wrist joint is rarely dislocated, but often sprained. It can be difficult to distinguish between a sprained and fractured wrist, especially if the scaphoid bone is injured.

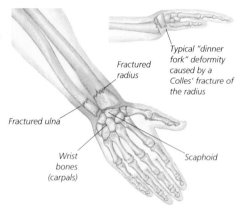

Typical "dinner fork" deformity caused by a Colles' fracture of the radius

Fractured radius

Fractured ulna

Wrist bones (carpals)

Scaphoid

TREATMENT

YOUR AIMS ARE:
- To immobilise the arm.
- To arrange removal to hospital.

1 Sit the casualty down. Gently steady and support the injured forearm across her chest. If necessary, carefully expose and treat any wound (*see page 142*).

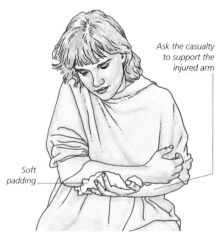

Ask the casualty to support the injured arm

Soft padding

2 Gently surround and cradle the forearm in folds of soft padding.

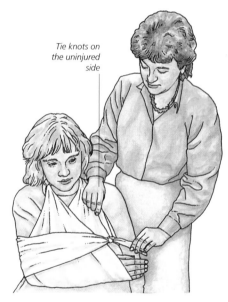

Tie knots on the uninjured side

3 Support the arm in an arm sling (*see page 214*). You may, if necessary, secure the limb to her chest, using a broad–fold bandage tied over the sling close to the elbow. Tie the knot in front, on the uninjured side.

4 Take or send the casualty to hospital, transporting in the sitting position.

INJURIES TO THE HAND AND FINGERS

The hand is made up of many small bones with movable joints, any one of which may be injured by direct or indirect force.

Multiple fractures affecting all of the hand are usually caused by crushing injuries, and there may be severe bleeding and swelling. Minor fractures are usually caused by direct force. The most common injury is a fracture of the knuckle between the little finger and the hand, which often results from a misplaced punch!

Dislocations and sprains may affect any of the fingers. The thumb is particularly prone to dislocation caused by a fall on to the hand (for example, while skiing).

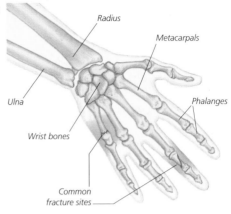

Radius

Metacarpals

Ulna

Phalanges

Wrist bones

Common fracture sites

TREATMENT

> YOUR AIMS ARE:
> • To immobilise and elevate the hand.
> • To arrange removal to hospital.

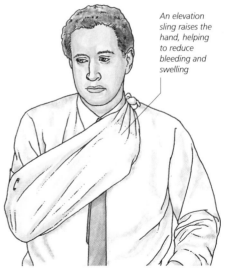

An elevation sling raises the hand, helping to reduce bleeding and swelling

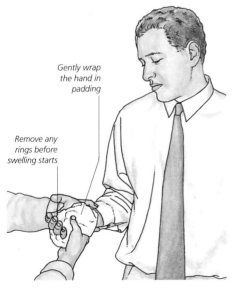

Gently wrap the hand in padding

Remove any rings before swelling starts

2 Gently support the affected arm in an elevation sling (see page 215).

3 You may, if necessary, secure the arm to the chest by applying a broad-fold bandage over the sling. Tie the knot in front on the uninjured side.

1 Protect the injured hand by surrounding it in folds of soft padding.

4 Take or send the casualty to hospital, transporting in the sitting position.

FRACTURES OF THE RIBCAGE

Rib fractures may be caused by direct force (a blow to, or fall on to, the chest), or by indirect force produced in a crush injury. If the fracture is complicated by a penetrating wound or a "flail chest" injury, breathing may be seriously impaired.

Flail chest injuries

If multiple rib fractures isolate a portion of the chest wall, this portion will move in when the casualty breathes in, and out when the casualty breathes out – the opposite of the normal chest movement. This state of "paradoxical breathing" produces severe respiratory difficulties.

RECOGNITION

Depending on severity, there may be:
- Sharp pain at the site of the fracture.
- Pain on taking a deep breath; the casualty's breathing may be shallow.
- Paradoxical breathing.
- An open wound over the fracture, through which you might hear air being "sucked" into the chest cavity.
- Features of internal bleeding (*see page 83*) and shock.

See also: Penetrating chest wounds, *page 88.*
Shock, *page 68.*

TREATMENT

YOUR AIMS ARE:
- To support the chest wall.
- To arrange removal to hospital.

FOR A FRACTURED RIB

Support the limb on the injured side in an arm sling (*see page 214*). Take or send the casualty to hospital.

FOR OPEN OR MULTIPLE FRACTURES

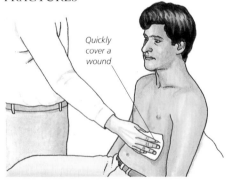

Quickly cover a wound

1 Immediately cover and seal any wounds to the chest wall.

2 Lay the casualty down. He may be most comfortable in a half-sitting position, with head and shoulders turned and body inclined towards the injured side. Support the limb on the injured side in an elevation sling (*see page 215*).

Elevation sling

Body inclined towards the injured side

IF the casualty becomes unconscious, or breathing becomes difficult and/or noisy, place him in the recovery position (*see page 30*), uninjured side uppermost.

3 Dial 999 for an ambulance.

BACK INJURIES

Possible injuries to the back include fractures of the bones of the spine, a displaced intervertebral disc ("slipped disc"), muscle strains, and ligament sprains. The chief danger with any back injury, but particularly fractures and disc injuries, is that the spinal cord or nerves may be damaged.

THE SPINE

The spine, or backbone, is actually made up of a column of small bones, each of which is called a *vertebra*. The spine supports the trunk and head, and surrounds and protects the spinal cord *(see page 114)*. The spinal column is supported by many strong ligaments and the muscles of the trunk.

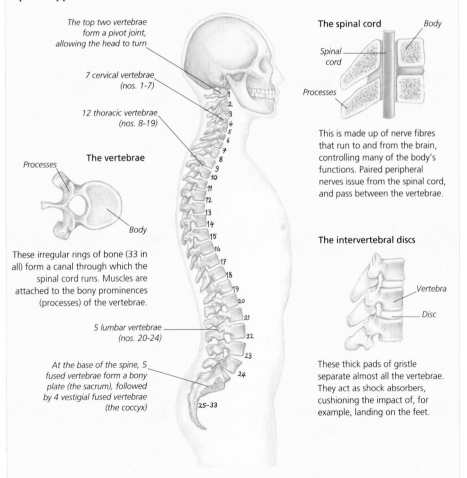

The top two vertebrae form a pivot joint, allowing the head to turn

7 cervical vertebrae (nos. 1-7)

12 thoracic vertebrae (nos. 8-19)

The vertebrae

Processes

Body

These irregular rings of bone (33 in all) form a canal through which the spinal cord runs. Muscles are attached to the bony prominences (processes) of the vertebrae.

5 lumbar vertebrae (nos. 20-24)

At the base of the spine, 5 fused vertebrae form a bony plate (the sacrum), followed by 4 vestigial fused vertebrae (the coccyx)

The spinal cord   Body

Spinal cord

Processes

This is made up of nerve fibres that run to and from the brain, controlling many of the body's functions. Paired peripheral nerves issue from the spinal cord, and pass between the vertebrae.

The intervertebral discs

Vertebra

Disc

These thick pads of gristle separate almost all the vertebrae. They act as shock absorbers, cushioning the impact of, for example, landing on the feet.

SPINAL INJURY

The danger of any spinal injury is that the spinal cord may be affected. The spinal cord is delicate and, if damaged, loss of power or sensation can occur in parts of the body below the injured area. Temporary damage can be caused if the cord or peripheral nerves are pinched by displaced discs or bone fragments; permanent damage will result if the cord is partially or completely severed.

Dangers of spinal fracture

Although the spinal cord may be injured without any damage to the bones, spinal fracture vastly increases the risk. Fractures of the vertebrae can be caused by both direct and indirect force. The most vulnerable parts of the spine are the bones in the neck and in the lower back.

What causes spinal injury?

Always suspect spinal injury when unusual or abnormal forces have been exerted on the back or neck, and particularly if the casualty complains of any disturbance of feeling or movement. The history of the injury is the most important indicator. If the casualty or witnesses tell you that the accident involved a violent forward bending, a backward bending, or a twisting injury of the spine, you must treat as for a fractured spine.

Possible causes of spinal injury

• Falling from a height.
• Falling awkwardly at gymnastics or trampolining.
• Diving into a shallow pool.
• Being thrown from a horse or from a motorbike.
• Collapse of a scrum at rugby.
• Sudden deceleration in a motor vehicle (for example, a head-on crash).
• A heavy object falling across the back.
• Injury to the head or face.

RECOGNITION

When only the spinal column is damaged, there may be:

• Pain in the neck or back at the level of the injury. This may be masked by other, more painful injuries.
• A step or twist in the normal curve of the spine.
• Tenderness on gently feeling the spine.

When the spinal cord has also been damaged, there may be:

• Loss of control over limbs. Movement may be weak or absent.
• Loss of sensation.
• Abnormal sensations – for example, burning or tingling. The casualty may tell you that limbs feel "stiff", "heavy", or "clumsy".
• Difficulty with breathing.

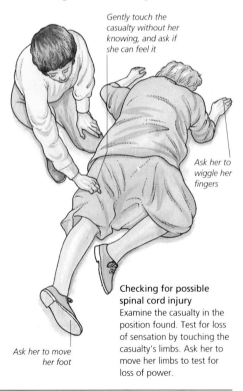

Gently touch the casualty without her knowing, and ask if she can feel it

Ask her to wiggle her fingers

Ask her to move her foot

Checking for possible spinal cord injury
Examine the casualty in the position found. Test for loss of sensation by touching the casualty's limbs. Ask her to move her limbs to test for loss of power.

TREATMENT FOR A CONSCIOUS CASUALTY

YOUR AIMS ARE:
- To prevent further injury.
- To arrange urgent removal to hospital.

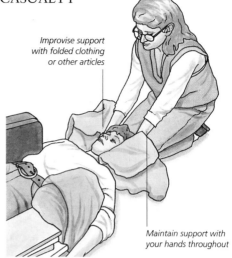

Improvise support with folded clothing or other articles

DO NOT move the casualty from the position found, unless she is in danger or becomes unconscious (*see overleaf*). If she must be moved, use a scoop stretcher (*see page 225*), or a modified log-roll (*see overleaf*).

1 Reassure the casualty, and tell her not to move.

Maintain support with your hands throughout

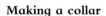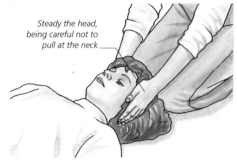

Steady the head, being careful not to pull at the neck

2 Steady and support her head in the neutral position by placing your hands over her ears. Maintain this support.

IF you suspect neck injury, get a helper to place rolled blankets or other articles around the casualty's neck and shoulders.

3 Dial 999 for an ambulance.

IF arrival of the ambulance is imminent, maintain support with your hands until it arrives.

IF removal is delayed you may, if the neck is injured, apply a collar. You *must* continue to hold the head and neck while, and after, the collar is fitted.

Making a collar

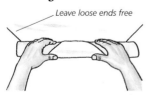

Leave loose ends free

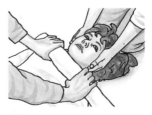

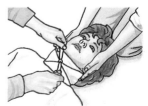

1 Fold a newspaper and wrap it in a triangular bandage or scarf, or insert it into a stocking or leg of a pair of tights.

2 Bend the wrapped newspaper over your thigh. Position the centre of the collar at the front of the casualty's neck, below the chin.

3 Pass the loose ends around the casualty's neck and tie in position at the front. Ensure that breathing is not impeded.

TREATMENT FOR AN UNCONSCIOUS CASUALTY

Check breathing and pulse. Positioning the casualty to resuscitate or protect the airway takes precedence over the injury.
• If breathing and pulse are present, place the casualty in a modified recovery position (*see opposite*), then dial 999.
• If pulse and breathing are absent, dial 999 for an ambulance and position the casualty to resuscitate as below.

YOUR AIMS ARE:
• To resuscitate the casualty, if necessary.
• To maintain an open airway.
• To prevent further damage to the spine or spinal cord.
• To arrange urgent removal to hospital.

IF BREATHING AND PULSE ARE ABSENT

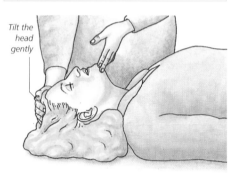

Tilt the head gently

1 Open and, if necessary, clear the airway. Tilt the head and lift the chin more gently than usual so that the head and neck remain in the neutral position.

2 Check breathing and pulse again. If they have not returned, combine artificial ventilation with chest compressions (*see page 38*) until help arrives.

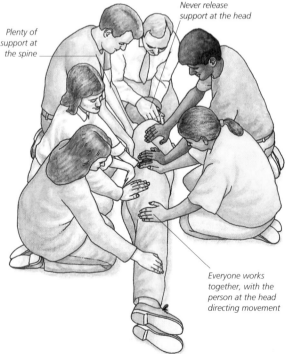

Never release support at the head

Plenty of support at the spine

Everyone works together, with the person at the head directing movement

IF you have to turn the casualty on to her back to resuscitate, you should keep head, trunk and toes in a straight line. While you maintain support at the neck, ask helpers (ideally five) to gently straighten the casualty's limbs, and "log-roll" her over. You can use the same technique to roll the casualty on to a stretcher.

THE RECOVERY POSITION IN SPINAL INJURY

If the casualty is unconscious with breathing and pulse present, you must place him in the recovery position (*see page 30*). With spinal injuries, you should, ideally, modify the position in order to keep the casualty's head and trunk aligned at all times. You will need at least one helper to do this successfully (*as shown below*); use more if you have them, but remember that even if you are alone with the casualty, he must be turned in order to protect the airway.

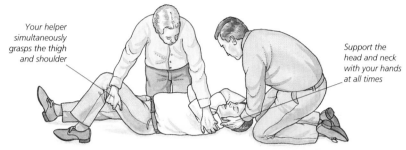

Your helper simultaneously grasps the thigh and shoulder

Support the head and neck with your hands at all times

1 Steady and support the casualty's head by placing your hands over his ears. Be prepared to maintain this support throughout, until help arrives.

2 Ask your helper to straighten the casualty's legs, and bring the arm nearest to him out, elbow bent, palm uppermost, at right-angles to the body.

3 Your helper grasps the casualty's thigh, drawing up the knee; then, bringing the casualty's other arm across his chest, grasps the far shoulder.

4 As he pulls the casualty towards him, you control the neutral position of the head and neck.

> DO NOT pull on the neck.

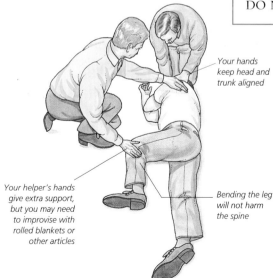

Your hands keep head and trunk aligned

Your helper's hands give extra support, but you may need to improvise with rolled blankets or other articles

Bending the leg will not harm the spine

5 Once the casualty is fully turned on to his side, both you and, if possible, your helper should support the casualty in this position until help arrives.

IF you have to send your helper to summon aid, rolled blankets, coats, or other articles may be placed alongside the casualty to keep him steady.

IF the injury is to the neck, a collar may be applied for further support (*see page 155*). This is *not* a substitute for support by the hands.

BACK PAIN

The lower back and neck are the most common sites of muscle strain or ligament sprain. In these areas, damage to intervertebral discs may irritate or pinch the spinal cord, or adjoining nerve roots.

How back pain is caused

Back and neck strain can be caused by prolonged bending, by lifting heavy weights, by strenuous exercise, or by an awkward fall. Neck sprain may be caused by the "whiplash" effect produced in a car accident. Other causes of backache include kidney disease, pregnancy, and menstruation.

Dangerous complications

If back pain is complicated by muscle spasms, fever, headache, nausea, vomiting, impaired consciousness, incontinence, or loss of sensation or movement, the casualty needs urgent hospital treatment.

RECOGNITION

There may be:
- Dull or severe pain in the back or neck, usually increased by movement.
- Pain travelling down any of the limbs, possibly with tingling and numbness.
- Spasm of the muscles, causing the neck or back to be held rigid or bent.
- Tenderness in the muscles.

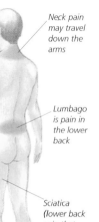

Neck pain may travel down the arms

Lumbago is pain in the lower back

Sciatica (lower back pain that "shoots" down the back of the leg) is caused by a trapped nerve

TREATMENT

YOUR AIMS ARE:
- To relieve pain.
- To seek medical aid if necessary.

FOR MINOR BACK PAIN

She may be more comfortable without a pillow

For severe back pain

Help the casualty to lie down as below, and call a doctor. If the pain is in the neck, a collar (*see page 155*) may provide relief. If there are complications, or you are worried about the casualty's condition, dial 999 for an ambulance.

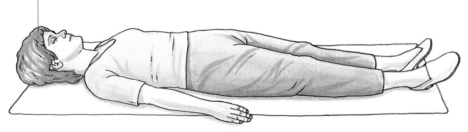

1 Help the casualty to lie down in the most comfortable position, either on the ground or on a firm mattress.

2 Advise the casualty to rest until the pain eases, and to see her doctor if symptoms persist.

FRACTURED PELVIS

Injuries to the pelvis are usually caused by crushing, or by indirect force, such as might occur in a car crash. The impact of a car dashboard on a knee can force the head of the thigh bone through the hip socket.

Pelvic injuries may be complicated by injury to internal tissues and organs, particularly the bladder and urinary passages, which the pelvis protects. Because of the bulk of body tissue surrounding the pelvis, internal bleeding may be severe, and shock often develops.

RECOGNITION

There may be:

* Inability to walk or even stand, although the legs appear sound.
* Pain and tenderness in the region of the hip, groin, or back, increased when the casualty moves.
* Blood at the urinary orifice, especially in a male casualty. The casualty may not be able to pass urine, or may find this painful.
* Signs of internal bleeding (*page 83*) and shock.

See also: Shock, *page 68*.

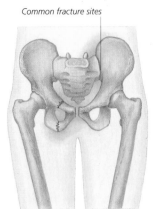

Common fracture sites

The pelvic girdle
This consists of three paired bones (the *ischium*, the *ilium* and the *pubis*) which are fused together.

TREATMENT

YOUR AIM IS:
* To arrange urgent removal to hospital.

DO NOT bandage the legs together if this causes intolerable pain.

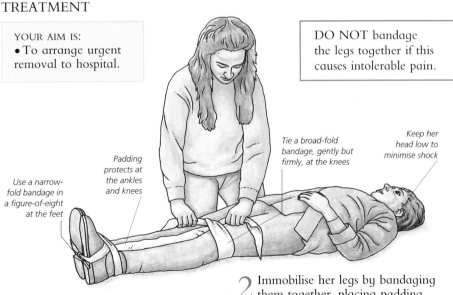

Use a narrow-fold bandage in a figure-of-eight at the feet

Padding protects at the ankles and knees

Tie a broad-fold bandage, gently but firmly, at the knees

Keep her head low to minimise shock

1 Help the casualty to lie on her back with her legs straight – or, if it is more comfortable for her, bend her knees slightly and support them.

2 Immobilise her legs by bandaging them together, placing padding between bony points.

3 Dial 999 for an ambulance. Treat the casualty for shock.

INJURIES TO THE LOWER LIMB

Injuries that may affect the lower limb, from the hip joint to the toes, include fractures, dislocations, sprains, and strains. It is important that casualties with lower limb injuries do not put weight on the injured leg.

INJURIES TO THE HIP AND THIGH

Fractures of the neck of the thigh bone (*femur*) at the hip joint are common in the elderly, and more frequent in women, whose bones become more porous and brittle as they age. This can be a stable injury; the casualty may be able to walk around for some time before the fracture is discovered. The hip may also, more rarely, be dislocated.

It takes considerable force (such as in road accidents, or falls from heights) to fracture the shaft of the thigh bone. This is a serious injury because, in most cases, a large volume of blood is lost into the tissues. This may cause shock to develop.

RECOGNITION

There may be:

• Pain at the site of the injury.
• Inability to walk.
• Signs of shock.
• Shortening of the thigh, as powerful muscles pull broken bone ends together.
• A turning outwards of the knee and foot.

See also: Shock, page 68.

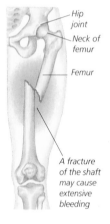

Hip joint

Neck of femur

Femur

A fracture of the shaft may cause extensive bleeding

TREATMENT

YOUR AIMS ARE:
• To immobilise the lower limb.
• To arrange urgent removal to hospital.

Pull the ankle firmly and steadily away from the knee

Maintain support at the injury while gentle traction is applied at the ankle

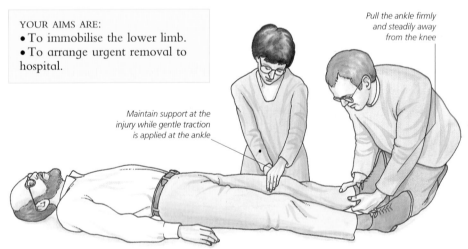

1 Lay the casualty down gently. Ask a helper to steady and support the injured limb.

2 Gently straighten the lower leg and apply traction at the ankle, pulling steadily in the line of the limb.

3 Dial 999 for an ambulance. If the ambulance will arrive quickly, support the leg with your hands until it arrives.

4 Take any steps possible to treat the casualty for shock; insulate him from the cold, but do not raise his legs.

IF the ambulance will be delayed, immobilise the limb by splinting it to the uninjured limb.

• Gently bring the casualty's sound limb alongside the injured one.

• Maintaining traction at the ankle, gently slide two bandages under the knees. Ease them into position above and below the fracture by sliding them backwards and forwards. Position another bandage at the knees and one at the ankles.

• Insert padding between the thighs, knees, and ankles, to prevent bandage-tying displacing the broken bone.

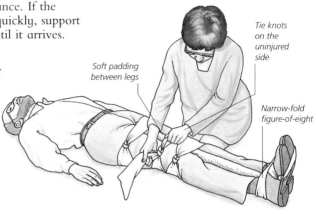

Tie knots on the uninjured side

Soft padding between legs

Narrow-fold figure-of-eight

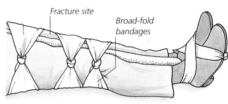

Fracture site

Broad-fold bandages

• Tie the bandages around his ankles and knees. Then tie the bandages above and below the fracture site.

To transport the casualty over a distance

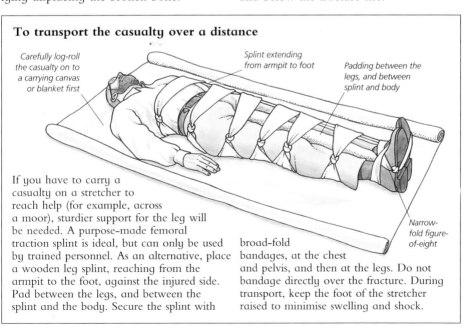

Carefully log-roll the casualty on to a carrying canvas or blanket first

Splint extending from armpit to foot

Padding between the legs, and between splint and body

Narrow-fold figure-of-eight

If you have to carry a casualty on a stretcher to reach help (for example, across a moor), sturdier support for the leg will be needed. A purpose-made femoral traction splint is ideal, but can only be used by trained personnel. As an alternative, place a wooden leg splint, reaching from the armpit to the foot, against the injured side. Pad between the legs, and between the splint and the body. Secure the splint with broad-fold bandages, at the chest and pelvis, and then at the legs. Do not bandage directly over the fracture. During transport, keep the foot of the stretcher raised to minimise swelling and shock.

INJURIES TO THE KNEE JOINT

The knee is the strong hinge joint between the thigh bone (*femur*) and shin bone (*tibia*). It is capable of bending, straightening, and, in the bent position, slight rotation. The knee joint is supported by strong muscles and ligaments, and protected in front by a disc of bone, the kneecap (*patella*). Any of these structures may be damaged by direct blows, violent twists, or strains.

RECOGNITION

There may be:
• History of a recent twist or blow to the knee.
• Pain, spreading from the injury to become deep-seated in the joint.
• If the bent knee has "locked", acute pain on attempting to straighten the leg.
• Rapid swelling at the knee joint.

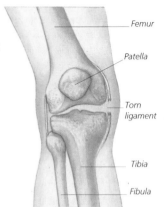

Femur

Patella

Torn ligament

Tibia

Fibula

TREATMENT

> YOUR AIMS ARE:
> • To protect the knee in the most comfortable position.
> • To arrange removal to hospital.

DO NOT attempt to force the knee straight. Displaced cartilage or internal bleeding may make the joint impossible to straighten safely.

DO NOT give the casualty anything to eat or drink; she may need to be given an anaesthetic.

DO NOT let the casualty walk.

1 Help the casualty to lie down, supporting her leg and knee in the most comfortable position.

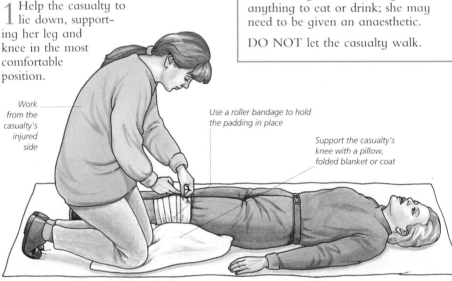

Work from the casualty's injured side

Use a roller bandage to hold the padding in place

Support the casualty's knee with a pillow, folded blanket or coat

2 Wrap soft padding around the joint, and bandage it carefully in place.

3 Take or send the casualty to hospital, transporting as a stretcher case.

INJURIES TO THE LOWER LEG

The sturdy shin bone (*tibia*) of the lower leg usually requires a heavy blow to break it (for example, from the bumper of a moving vehicle).

The thinner splint bone (*fibula*) can be broken by the type of twisting injury that sprains the ankle. Because the load-bearing shin bone remains intact, the casualty may be able to walk, and may be unaware that a fracture has occurred.

RECOGNITION

There will be:
• Localised pain.

There may be:
• A recent blow or wrench of the foot.
• An open wound.
• Inability to walk.

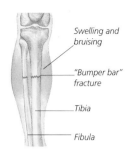

Swelling and bruising

"Bumper bar" fracture

Tibia

Fibula

TREATMENT

YOUR AIMS ARE:
• To immobilise the leg.
• To arrange urgent removal to hospital.

2 Straighten the leg using traction, pulling gently in the line of the shin.

3 Dial 999 for an ambulance. If the ambulance will arrive quickly, support the leg with your hands until it arrives.

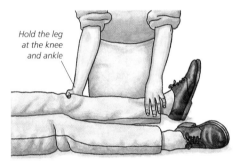

Hold the leg at the knee and ankle

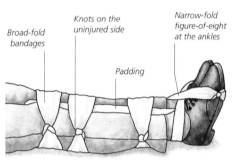

Broad-fold bandages

Knots on the uninjured side

Narrow-fold figure-of-eight at the ankles

Padding

1 Help the casualty to lie down, and carefully steady and support the injured leg. If necessary, gently expose and treat any wound (*see page 142*).

To transport the casualty

If you have to transport the casualty on a stretcher, place extra padding (for example, rolled blankets) on either side of the legs, from the upper thigh to the foot. Secure with broad-fold bandages at the thigh and knee, and above and below the fracture. Tie a figure-of-eight around the feet and ankles with a narrow-fold bandage.

IF the ambulance will be delayed, splint the injured limb to the sound one.
• Gently bring the sound limb alongside the injured one.
• Maintaining support at the ankle, gently slide bandages under the knees and ankles. Position them above and below the fracture, and at knees and ankles, avoiding the fracture if it is close to a joint.
• Insert padding between the knees and ankles, and between the calves.
• Tie the bandages around ankles and knees, then above and below the fracture. Bandage firmly, but avoid jerky movements.

SPRAINED ANKLE

While a broken ankle should be treated as a fracture of the lower leg (*see page 163*), a sprain (usually caused by a wrench) can be treated by the RICE procedure (*see also page 143*).

RECOGNITION

There will be:
- Pain, increased by movement or by putting weight on the foot.
- Swelling.

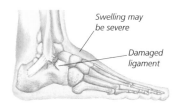

Swelling may be severe

Damaged ligament

TREATMENT

> YOUR AIMS ARE:
> - To relieve pain and swelling.
> - To seek medical aid if necessary.

1 Rest, steady, and support the ankle in the most comfortable position.

2 Cool a recent injury to reduce swelling, by applying an ice pack or cold compress (*see page 203*).

3 Wrap the ankle in a thick layer of padding, and bandage firmly.

4 Raise and support the injured limb.

5 Advise the casualty to rest the ankle, and to see his doctor if pain persists.

IF you suspect a broken bone, secure and support it as on page 163, and take or send the casualty to hospital.

FRACTURES OF THE FOOT

Fractures affecting the many small bones of the foot are usually caused by crushing injuries. These fractures are best treated at hospital.

RECOGNITION

There may be:
- Difficulty in walking.
- Stiffness of movement.
- Bruising and swelling.

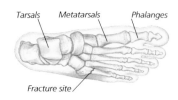

Tarsals   Metatarsals   Phalanges

Fracture site

TREATMENT

> YOUR AIMS ARE:
> - To minimise swelling.
> - To arrange removal to hospital.

1 Raise and support the foot to minimise swelling.

2 Apply an ice pack or cold compress (*see page 203*).

3 Take or send the casualty to hospital, keeping the foot elevated.

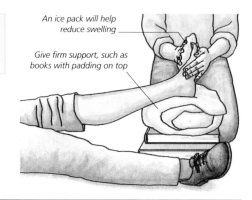

An ice pack will help reduce swelling

Give firm support, such as books with padding on top

POISONING

P oisoning is often accidental, involving substances in everyday use, but can also be deliberate (for example, in cases of attempted suicide).
It can occur in the home or the workplace as a
result of accidents, or be caused by eating
contaminated food or poisonous plants. Drugs and
alcohol, if misused, can also poison the body.

Recognising and treating poisoning

Features of poisoning vary depending on the
poison, the method of entry, and the amount
taken. A conscious casualty or an onlooker may
tell you that poisoning has occurred. If the
casualty is unconscious, external features (such as
a fume-filled room or a suspect container) may
tell you what you need to know.

Medical attention is always advisable in cases of
poisoning, and is essential in severe cases, when
the First Aider may have to act swiftly to preserve
life. Although poisoning can be fatal, most cases
are successfully treated. It will help the doctor in
treatment if you can identify the poison involved.

CONTENTS

THE FIRST AIDER SHOULD:

• If the casualty is unconscious, ensure an open
airway, and monitor breathing and circulation.

• Prevent further injury:
FOR SWALLOWED POISONS: do not attempt to induce
vomiting, as this may harm the casualty further.
FOR INHALED POISONS: remove the casualty from
danger and into fresh air.
FOR ABSORBED POISONS: flush away any residual
chemical on the skin.

• Obtain appropriate medical attention.

WHAT IS A POISON?

A poison (or *toxin*) is a substance which, if taken into the body in sufficient quantity, can cause temporary or permanent damage. Poisons may be swallowed, inhaled, absorbed through the skin, *instilled* at the eye, or injected.

Once in the body, poisons may work their way into the bloodstream, and be swiftly carried to all the tissues. Signs and symptoms vary depending on the poison and its method of entry, though vomiting is common to many cases, with the risk to the casualty that stomach contents may be inhaled.

The digestive system

The body "processes" food to extract its nutrients and eliminate waste that includes many mildly toxic elements. From the stomach, food passes into the small intestine, where nutrients are broken down and absorbed into the blood. This blood then filters through the liver, which inactivates many toxins. The kidneys also filter and excrete impurities. The food residue passes to the large intestine, and waste is expelled at the anus.

How poisons enter the body

Poisons may enter at the eye, possibly causing chemical burns

Poisonous gases, solvents, vapours or fumes may be inhaled

Swallowed poisons may enter the circulatory system through the walls of the digestive tract

Injected poisons and drugs enter the bloodstream rapidly. Poisonous snakes, fish or insects may inject their venom into the skin. Dangerous drugs, particularly narcotics, are injected by abusers

Liver

Kidneys

Strong chemicals, such as corrosives and pesticides, may be absorbed through the skin, and may also cause burns

Small intestine

How poisons affect the body

Poisons reaching the brain may cause confusion, delirium, fits, and unconsciousness

Swallowed corrosives can burn the lips, mouth, and food passages

Inhaled poisons can cause severe respiratory distress

Some poisons disturb the action of the heart

The body's poison filters, the liver and kidneys, can be seriously damaged by an "overload" of toxins

Stomach

Poison in the digestive system can cause vomiting, abdominal pain, and diarrhoea

Poisons may damage the blood itself, preventing the red cells from carrying oxygen to the tissues

Large intestine

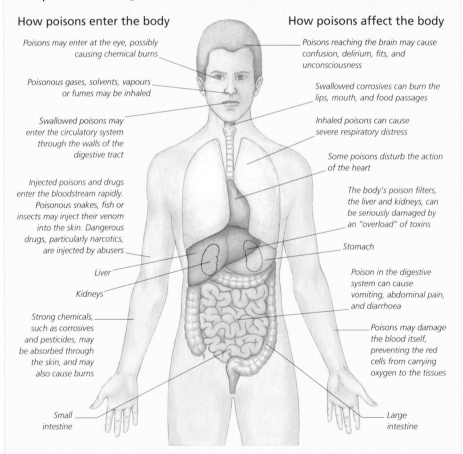

HOUSEHOLD POISONS

Almost every household contains poison-ous substances, such as bleach, paint strip-per, glue, paraffin, and weedkiller, which can be spilled, causing chemical burns, or swallowed. Children in particular are at risk from accidental household poisoning.

See also: Chemical burns, *page 110.*
Drug poisoning, *page 168.*
Inhalation of fumes, *page 60.*
Unconsciousness, *page 115.*

Preventing poisoning in the home
• Keep dangerous chemicals out of children's reach (*not* under the sink).
• Keep medicines in a locked cupboard.
• Leave poisonous household substances in their original containers – never put them in old soft-drinks bottles.
• Buy medicines and household sub-stances in tamper-proof containers.

TREATMENT

YOUR AIMS ARE:
• To maintain airway, breathing, and circulation.
• To obtain medical aid.
• To identify the poison.

FOR CHEMICALS ON THE SKIN

1 Wash away any residual chemical on the skin with plenty of water.

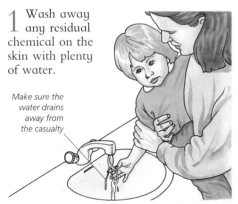

Make sure the water drains away from the casualty

DO NOT contaminate yourself with the dangerous chemical or the rinsing water.

---

2 Use your judgement to call a doctor or dial 999 for an ambulance. Give information about the spilled chemical.

FOR SWALLOWED POISONS

1 Check and, if necessary, clear the airway.

The recovery position lessens the risks of vomiting

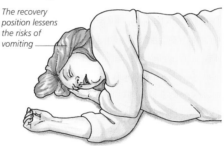

IF the casualty is unconscious, check breathing and pulse, and be prepared to resuscitate. If artificial ventilation is necessary, a plastic face shield will protect you if there is burning around the mouth. Place the casualty in the recovery pos-ition (*see page 30*); she may well vomit.

DO NOT try to induce vomiting.

---

2 Use your judgement to call a doctor or dial 999 for an ambulance. Give information about the swallowed poison.

IF a conscious casualty's lips are burned by corrosive substances, give her fre-quent sips of cold water or milk.

DRUG POISONING

This can result from an accidental or deliberate overdose of prescribed or over-the-counter drugs, or from active drug abuse. The features of drug poisoning vary depending on the drug taken and the method of entry (*see below*).

See also: Unconsciousness, *page 115*.

DRUG	EFFECTS
Painkillers Aspirin (commonly swallowed)	Upper abdominal pain, nausea, and vomiting (possibly blood-stained) • Ringing in the ears • "Sighing" breathing • Confusion or delirium
Paracetamol (commonly swallowed)	Little effect at first. Later, features of liver damage: upper abdominal pain and tenderness, nausea, and vomiting
Nervous system depressants – barbiturates and tranquillisers (commonly swallowed)	Lethargy and sleepiness, leading to unconsciousness • Shallow breathing • A weak, irregular, or abnormally slow or fast pulse
Stimulants and hallucinogens – amphetamines and LSD (commonly swallowed); cocaine (commonly inhaled)	Excitable, hyperactive behaviour, wildness and frenzy • Sweating • Tremor of the hands • Hallucinations: the casualty may be "hearing" voices, and/or "seeing" things
Narcotics – morphine, heroin (commonly injected)	Constricted pupils • Sluggishness and confusion, possibly leading to unconsciousness • Slow, shallow breathing, which may cease • Needle marks may be infected, or infection may be introduced by dirty needles
Solvents (commonly inhaled) – glue, lighter fuel	Nausea, vomiting, and headaches • Hallucinations • Possibly, unconsciousness • Rarely, cardiac arrest

TREATMENT

YOUR AIMS ARE:
• To maintain airway, breathing, and circulation.
• To arrange urgent removal to hospital.

1 Check and, if necessary, clear the airway.

IF the casualty is unconscious, check for breathing and a pulse.

2 Place the casualty in the recovery position (*see page 30*).

DO NOT attempt to induce vomiting. It is often ineffective, and may harm the casualty further.

3 Dial 999 for an ambulance. Preserve samples of vomited material, empty containers, or "suicide" notes. Send these with the casualty to hospital.

INDUSTRIAL POISONS

Poisoning can occur in the workplace as a result of a leak, failure of a chemical plant, or a major accident. Most cases of industrial poisoning involve poisonous gases. Spillage of corrosive chemicals can also result in burns. Factories using potentially dangerous gases or chemicals may keep oxygen equipment, and must display notices indicating action to be taken in cases of emergency. Workers should be familiar with such advice.

See also: Chemical burns, *page 110.*
Inhalation of fumes, *page 60.*
Hazardous substances, *page 19.*
Unconsciousness, *page 115.*

TREATMENT

YOUR AIMS ARE:
• To remove the casualty from danger *without* endangering yourself.
• To arrange urgent removal to hospital.

FOR INHALED GASES

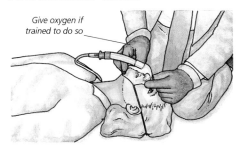

Give oxygen if trained to do so

1 If possible, remove the casualty from danger and into fresh air. Dial 999 for an ambulance. Administer oxygen if you have been trained in its use.

DO NOT enter a gas-filled room unless you are authorised and properly equipped to do so.

IF the casualty is unconscious, check breathing and pulse, and be prepared to resuscitate if necessary.

2 Place the casualty in the recovery position (*see page 30*).

FOR CHEMICALS ON THE SKIN

1 Flush away any residual chemical on the skin with plenty of cold water.

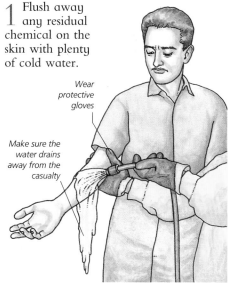

Wear protective gloves

Make sure the water drains away from the casualty

DO NOT contaminate yourself with the dangerous chemical or the rinsing water.

2 Dial 999 for an ambulance.

IF he becomes unconscious, check breathing and pulse, and be prepared to resuscitate (using, if necessary, a plastic face shield). Place him in the recovery position.

ALCOHOL POISONING

Alcohol (*ethanol*) is a drug that depresses the activity of the central nervous system. Small quantities generally produce only a slight change of mood. Prolonged intake can result in all physical and mental abilities becoming severely impaired, and deep unconsciousness can ensue.

Dangers of alcohol poisoning

• An unconscious casualty is in danger of inhaling and choking on vomit.
• Because alcohol dilates the blood vessels, hypothermia may develop if the casualty is exposed to the cold.
• A casualty with head injuries who smells of alcohol may be misdiagnosed.

RECOGNITION

There may be:
• A strong smell of alcohol.
• Unconsciousness. The casualty may be rousable, but will quickly relapse.
• A flushed and moist face.
• Deep, noisy breathing.
• A full, bounding pulse.

In the later stages of unconsciousness:
• A dry, bloated appearance to the face.
• Shallow breathing.
• Dilated pupils that react poorly to light.
• A weak, rapid pulse.

See also: Hypothermia, *page 130.*
Drunkenness, *page 126.*

TREATMENT

YOUR AIMS ARE:
• To maintain an open airway.
• To seek appropriate medical attention.

IF the casualty is unresponsive, check breathing and pulse, and be prepared to resuscitate if necessary. Place him in the recovery position (*see page 30*).

2 Use your judgement to call a doctor or dial 999 for an ambulance.

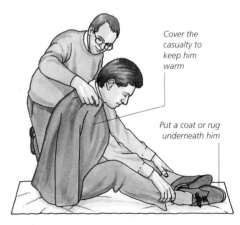

Shake and shout: "Can you hear me?" or "Open your eyes!"

Cover the casualty to keep him warm

Put a coat or rug underneath him

1 Check the casualty's level of response. Carefully shake his shoulders and shout at him to see if he responds.

3 Protect the casualty from the cold; insulate him from the ground, and cover with a coat or blanket.

POISONOUS PLANTS

Although there are relatively few poisonous plants in the United Kingdom, they can cause serious illness if eaten. Young children are most at risk, as they are attracted to brightly coloured berries and seeds, and are liable to eat them.

See also: Unconsciousness, *page 115.*

PLANTS THAT ARE POISONOUS IF SWALLOWED

Mushrooms	Seeds, bulbs, and rhizomes	Berries
Death cap Brown roll rim Spotted fly agaric *Cortinarius speciosissimus* (often mistaken for the edible chanterelle)	Laburnum Lupin Daffodil Iris	Deadly nightshade Holly Laurel Mistletoe Yew Wild arum (lords-and-ladies)

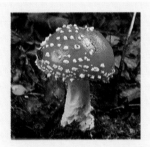

Fly agaric (*Amanita muscari*)

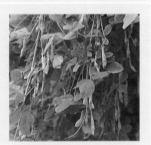

Laburnum seed pods

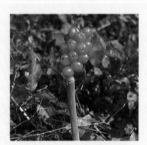

Wild arum (*Arum maculatum*)

TREATMENT

YOUR AIMS ARE:
• To maintain airway, breathing, and circulation.
• To obtain medical aid.

DO NOT try to induce vomiting. It is often ineffective, and may harm the casualty further.

1 Check and, if necessary, clear the airway.

IF the casualty is unconscious, check breathing and pulse, and be prepared to resuscitate if necessary. Place the casualty in the recovery position (*see page 30*); he or she may well vomit.

2 Use your judgement to call a doctor or dial 999 for an ambulance. If in doubt, always call an ambulance.

3 Try to identify the plant, and which part of it has been eaten. Preserve pieces of the plant, and samples of any vomited material, to show the doctor or send with the casualty to hospital.

FOOD POISONING

This may be caused by eating food that is contaminated, either by bacteria or by toxins produced by bacteria that were present in the food at some stage.

Types of food poisoning

Bacterial food poisoning is often caused by the *salmonella* group of bacteria (associated with farm animals, particularly poultry). Symptoms may appear within a few hours, or be delayed for a day or so.

Toxic food poisoning is frequently caused by toxins produced by the bacteria group *staphylococcus*. Symptoms usually develop rapidly – possibly within two to six hours of consumption.

Preventing food poisoning

• Ensure that frozen meat and poultry are fully defrosted before cooking.
• Cook meat, poultry, and eggs thoroughly to destroy dangerous bacteria.
• Never keep food lukewarm for long periods; it allows bacteria to multiply without any obvious signs of spoilage.
• Ensure hands are clean before preparing food. Wear protective gloves if you have any wounds on your hands.

RECOGNITION

There may be:
• Nausea and vomiting.
• Cramping abdominal pains.
• Diarrhoea (possibly bloodstained).
• Headache.
• Fever.
• Features of shock.
• Collapse.

See also: Diarrhoea and vomiting, page 184.
Shock, page 68.

TREATMENT

YOUR AIMS ARE:
• To make the casualty rest.
• To seek medical advice or aid.

1 Help the casualty to lie down and rest.

2 Call a doctor.

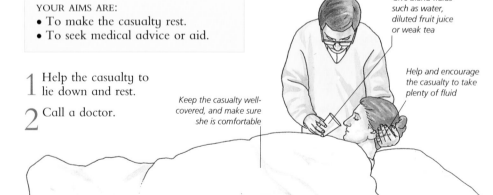

Give bland fluids such as water, diluted fruit juice or weak tea

Help and encourage the casualty to take plenty of fluid

Keep the casualty well-covered, and make sure she is comfortable

3 Give the casualty plenty to drink, and a bowl in case she vomits.

IF the casualty's condition worsens, dial 999 for an ambulance.

FOREIGN BODIES

The term "foreign body" is used to describe any extraneous material that finds its way into the body, either through a wound in the skin, or via one of the natural orifices of the body, such as the ear, nose, or mouth. Foreign bodies – commonly, specks of dirt or grit – can also rest on, or enter, the eye. Injuries in which a foreign body is a complication of a wound, or has entered an eye wound, are dealt with in the chapter *Wounds and Bleeding*, pages 75-96.

What you will find in this chapter

The pages that follow cover everyday incidents such as removing splinters and fish hooks from the skin, or particles floating on the surface of the eye. There is also advice on managing situations where objects have been swallowed, inhaled, or inserted into an ear or the nose. Objects that have, for whatever reason, found their way into the ano-genital orifices are not the concern of the First Aider, and should be referred to a doctor or nurse.

CONTENTS

THE FIRST AIDER SHOULD:

• Decide whether it is feasible or wise to attempt to remove the object. Certain foreign bodies cannot, or should not, be removed by the First Aider. If the object cannot be removed, obtain medical aid.

• If the foreign body can be removed, ensure that the casualty keeps still. Reassurance and, possibly, considerable firmness will be required.

• After removing the foreign body, take any necessary further steps; seek a doctor's advice if you suspect internal injury, or a risk of infection.

FOREIGN BODIES IN THE SKIN

Small foreign bodies (wood splinters, shards of glass) usually cause minor puncture wounds with little or no bleeding. If a portion of the object protrudes from the skin, you may attempt to draw it out. Foreign bodies deeply embedded in a wound should not be removed by a First Aider; you may cause further injury.

Foreign bodies are often contaminated with dirt and bacteria. Ensure that the wound is clean, and that the casualty's tetanus immunisation is up to date.

See also: Foreign bodies in minor wounds, *page 95.*
Infection in wounds, *page 96.*
Severe external bleeding, *page 78.*

SPLINTERS

Small splinters of wood, metal, or glass in the skin, particularly of the hands, feet, and knees, are common injuries. The splinter can usually be successfully drawn out using tweezers. However, if the splinter is deeply embedded, lies over a joint, or proves difficult to remove, it is better left alone until seen by a doctor.

TREATMENT

> YOUR AIMS ARE:
> • To remove the splinter.
> • To minimise the risk of infection.

1 Clean the area around the splinter with soap and warm water. Sterilize a pair of tweezers by passing them through a flame.

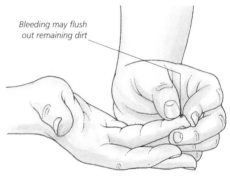

Bleeding may flush out remaining dirt

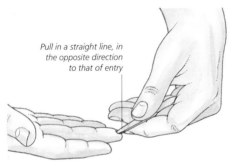

Pull in a straight line, in the opposite direction to that of entry

2 Grasp the splinter as close to the skin as possible, and draw it out along the track of its entry.

3 Squeeze the wound to encourage a little bleeding. Clean the area and apply an adhesive dressing ("plaster").

IF the splinter does not come out easily, or breaks up, treat as an embedded foreign body (*see page 95*). *Never* probe the area (for example, with a needle).

4 Check that the casualty's tetanus immunisation is up to date *(see page 96)*. If not, or if in doubt, advise the casualty to see her doctor.

FISH HOOKS

Embedded fish hooks are difficult to with-draw because of their barbs; you should only attempt removal if medical aid is not readily available. Advise the casualty to see a doctor after removal if tetanus immunity is in doubt (*see page 96*).

TREATMENT

> YOUR AIM IS:
> • To remove the hook, if possible, without causing further injury and pain.

WHEN MEDICAL AID IS AVAILABLE

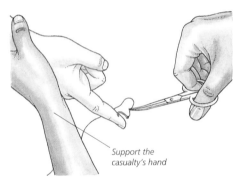

Support the casualty's hand

1 Cut the fishing line close to the hook.

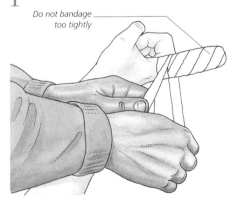

Do not bandage too tightly

2 Build up pads of gauze around the hook until you can bandage over it without pushing it in further. Ensure that the casualty receives medical attention.

WHEN MEDICAL AID IS NOT READILY AVAILABLE

If the barb is not visible

1 Loop a piece of fishing line around the curve of the hook.

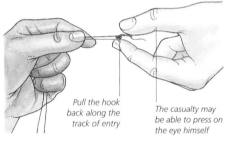

Pull the hook back along the track of entry

The casualty may be able to press on the eye himself

2 Pressing the eye of the hook down on the finger, pull sharply on the line to withdraw the hook. If the eye extends beyond the finger, pad under the shaft and press the eye down on the padding.

3 Clean and dress the wound. Ensure that tetanus immunity is up to date.

If the barb is visible

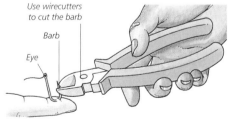

Use wirecutters to cut the barb

Barb

Eye

1 Cut the barb away, and carefully withdraw the hook by the eye.

2 Clean and dress the wound. Ensure that tetanus immunity is up to date.

FOREIGN BODIES IN THE EYE

A speck of dust or grit, or a loose eyelash floating on the white of the eye can generally be removed easily. However, a foreign body that adheres to the eye, penetrates the eyeball, or rests on the coloured part of the eye (the *pupil* and *iris*) should *not* be removed by a First Aider.

RECOGNITION

There may be:

- Blurred vision, pain, or discomfort.
- Redness and watering of the eye.
- Eyelids screwed up in spasm.

See also: Eye wounds, *page 91.*

TREATMENT

> YOUR AIM IS:
> - To prevent injury to the eye.

> DO NOT touch anything sticking to, or embedded in, the eyeball, or on the coloured part of the eye. Cover the affected eye with an eye pad, bandage both eyes, then take or send the casualty to hospital.

1 Advise the casualty not to rub her eye. Sit her down facing the light.

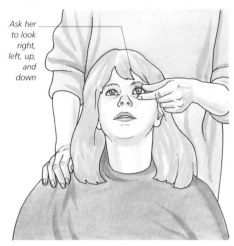

Ask her to look right, left, up, and down

2 Gently separate the eyelids with your finger and thumb. Examine every part of her eye.

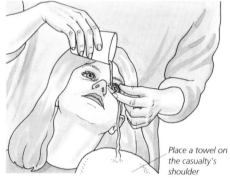

Place a towel on the casualty's shoulder

3 If you can see the foreign body, wash it out using a glass or an eye irrigator, and clean water (sterile, if possible).

4 If this is unsuccessful then, providing the foreign body is not stuck in place, lift it off with a moist swab, or the damp corner of a tissue or clean handkerchief.

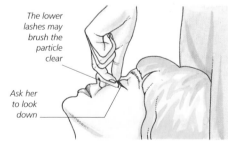

The lower lashes may brush the particle clear

Ask her to look down

IF the object is under the eyelid, grasping the lashes, pull the upper lid over the lower lid. Blinking the eye under water may also make the object float clear.

FOREIGN BODIES IN THE NOSE

Young children at the "exploring" age may push small objects up their noses. Sharp objects can damage the tissues of the nostrils, while smooth objects can cause blockage and infection. You must not try to extricate these items; you may cause injury or push the object in further. The casualty must be seen at hospital.

RECOGNITION

There may be:

- Difficulty in breathing, or noisy breathing, through the nose.
- Swelling of the nose.
- Smelly or blood-stained discharge may indicate an object present for some time.

TREATMENT

YOUR AIM IS:
• To obtain medical attention.

DO NOT attempt to remove the foreign body.

1 Keep the casualty quiet. Advise him or her to breathe through the mouth.

2 Take or send the casualty to hospital.

FOREIGN BODIES IN THE EAR

Small children often push objects into the ear which, if they become lodged, can cause temporary deafness by blocking the ear canal, or may damage the ear drum.

Pieces of cotton wool are sometimes left in the ear after cleaning. Occasionally, insects fly or crawl into the ear; their buzzing or movement may cause alarm.

TREATMENT

YOUR AIMS ARE:
• To prevent injury to the ear.
• To obtain medical aid if necessary.

FOR A LODGED FOREIGN BODY

DO NOT attempt to remove the object. You may cause serious injury, and push the foreign body in even further.

Take or send the casualty to hospital. Reassure the casualty during transport, or until help arrives.

FOR AN INSECT IN THE EAR

1 Sit the casualty down.

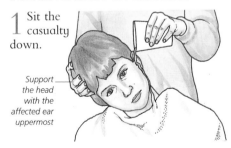

Support the head with the affected ear uppermost

2 Gently flood the ear with tepid water so that the insect floats out.

3 If this is unsuccessful, take or send the casualty to hospital.

SWALLOWED FOREIGN BODIES

Young children often put things in their mouths. Small objects such as coins, pins, or buttons can be swallowed. Sharp objects may damage the digestive tract; small, smooth objects are unlikely to cause injury, but can cause choking.

See also: Choking, *page 57.*

TREATMENT

YOUR AIM IS: • To obtain medical attention.	DO NOT give the casualty anything to eat or drink.

FOR SHARP OR LARGE OBJECTS

Dial 999 for an ambulance. Reassure the casualty while waiting for help to arrive.

FOR SMALL, SMOOTH OBJECTS

Reassure the casualty, and take or send him or her to hospital or to a doctor.

INHALED FOREIGN BODIES

Small, smooth objects can slip past the protective mechanisms within the throat and enter the air passages. Dry peanuts, which swell up when in contact with body fluids, pose a particular danger in young children as they can be inhaled into the lung, causing serious damage.

RECOGNITION

There may be:
• Some sign or noise of choking which quickly passes.
• A persistent dry cough.

See also: Choking, *page 57.*

TREATMENT

YOUR AIM IS: • To maintain an open airway.   • To obtain urgent medical attention.

1 Treat for choking if necessary.

2 Take or send the casualty to hospital.

3 Reassure the casualty during transport, or while waiting for the ambulance to arrive. Try to find out what it is that has been inhaled.

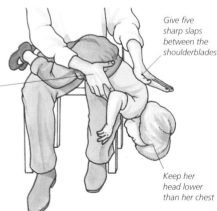

Give five sharp slaps between the shoulderblades

Put a choking child over your knee, and support her with one hand

Keep her head lower than her chest

MISCELLANEOUS CONDITIONS

T he boundary between first aid and home medicine is often not clear-cut. Many everyday conditions (for example, aches and pains, or a raised temperature) develop quickly and need prompt treatment. While some of the common ailments described in this chapter are not included in formal first aid training, they will nevertheless benefit from sensible first aid measures. Common sense and good preparation can also help to prevent and treat illness while travelling overseas.

The use of medicines

While this chapter describes the use of paracetamol and other tablets to relieve fever and pain, the giving of medication is not strictly within the scope of first aid, and should be supported by the advice of a doctor or pharmacist. More guidance is given on this subject, and on taking a casualty's temperature, in *Caring for the Sick,* this book's companion volume.

When to seek medical aid

An apparently trivial upset can sometimes be the start of serious illness. If you are in any doubt about your ability to deal with any of these conditions, you should always consult a doctor – even if only by telephone.

CONTENTS

THE FIRST AIDER SHOULD:

• Make the casualty as comfortable as possible.

• Take any possible steps to relieve pain and distress.

• If simple measures fail to provide relief within an hour or so, seek medical advice.

FEVER

A sustained body temperature above the normal level of 37°C (98.6°F) is known as fever, and is usually, though not always, caused by infection (by bacteria or viruses). Conditions associated with a high temperature include influenza ('flu), chicken pox, measles, meningitis, and local infections (for example, an abscess).

When to call a doctor

A moderate fever is not harmful, but a temperature of above 40°C (102°F) can be dangerous, and may trigger fits in infants and young children. Call a doctor, even if only for advice, if in doubt about the casualty's condition.

RECOGNITION
There will be:
- Raised under-the-tongue temperature.

In the early stages, there may be:
- Pallor.
- A "chilled" feeling – goose pimples, shivering, and chattering teeth.

As the fever advances, there may be:
- Hot, flushed skin, and sweating.
- Headache.
- Generalised "aches and pains".
- Raised armpit temperature.

See also: Heatstroke, *page 134.*
Convulsions in children, *page 122.*

TREATMENT

> YOUR AIMS ARE:
> - To make the casualty comfortable.
> - To bring down the fever.
> - To seek medical aid, if necessary.

1 Make the casualty comfortable in surroundings that are evenly warm, preferably in bed, and let her rest.

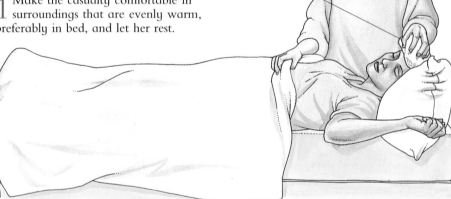

If the fever is very high, or if the casualty is a young child, cool by sponging with tepid water

2 Give the casualty plenty of bland fluids to drink. A small "hot toddy" may comfort an adult and may induce restful sleep. Give no more than one double measure of spirits.

3 An adult may take two paracetamol tablets. A child may be given the recommended dose of paracetamol syrup (*not* aspirin), and should be sponged with tepid water to lower the temperature.

HEADACHE

A headache may accompany any illness, particularly a feverish ailment such as 'flu, but may be the most prominent symptom of some serious condition (for example, meningitis or stroke). Mild "poisoning" by a stuffy or fume-filled atmosphere, or by unwise consumption of alcohol or other drugs, can induce a headache in an otherwise healthy person. Headaches may develop for no apparent reason, but can often be traced to tiredness, nervous tension, stress or emotional upset, or undue heat or cold.

Headaches range from constant low-grade discomfort to "blinding" pain that is completely incapacitating.

When to call a doctor

Always seek urgent advice if the pain:
• Develops very suddenly.
• Is severe and incapacitating.
• Is recurrent or persistent.
• Is accompanied by impaired consciousness, or loss of power or sensation.
• Is accompanied by a stiff neck.
• Follows a head injury.

TREATMENT

YOUR AIMS ARE:
• To relieve the pain.
• To seek medical aid if necessary.

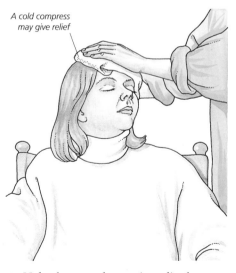

A cold compress may give relief

Migraine
Many people are prone to these severe, "sickening" headaches. They can be triggered by a variety of causes. Migraine sufferers usually recognise, and know best how to deal with, an attack. They may carry special medicines.

Migraines usually follow a pattern:
• There may be a warning period with disturbance of vision, in the form of flickering lights and/or a "blind patch".
• An intense throbbing headache, which may be one-sided, may develop.
• There may be discomfort in the upper abdomen, nausea, and vomiting.
• The casualty cannot tolerate any bright light or loud noise.

What you can do
Treatment is as for any headache, but help the casualty to take any special medication he or she may have (tablets or nasal sprays) and provide towels and a container in case he or she is sick.

1 Help the casualty to sit or lie down comfortably in a quiet place.

2 If possible, deal with any likely cause of the headache, such as loud noise, bright light, or lack of fresh air.

3 An adult may take two paracetamol tablets, or her own painkillers.

IF the pain does not ease within two hours, or if you are worried about the casualty's condition, call a doctor.

EARACHE

Earache, particularly in children, is most commonly due to an infection of the middle ear, and may be accompanied by a discharge. It can also accompany a cold, tonsillitis, measles, or 'flu. Pain may also be caused by a boil in the ear canal, a foreign body in the ear, or an abscess in a nearby tooth.

Earache caused by an infection is usually characterised by throbbing pain. A "steady" earache can also be caused by sudden changes in pressure in the middle ear (for example, during air travel).

Both types of earache may be accompanied by partial or total hearing loss on the affected side.

TREATMENT

YOUR AIMS ARE:
- To relieve pain.
- To obtain medical aid if necessary.

FOR THROBBING EARACHE

IF there is a discharge, fever, or marked hearing loss, call a doctor immediately.

1 A child with earache may be given the recommended dose of paracetamol syrup (*not* aspirin); an adult may take two paracetamol tablets, or her own painkillers.

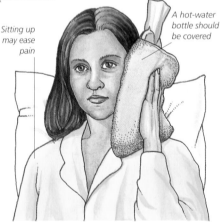

Sitting up may ease pain

A hot-water bottle should be covered

Pressure–change earache

Many people are prone to pressure-change earache on plane journeys. It may help to chew gum, or suck a sweet. (Remember that chewing gum should never be given to young children.)

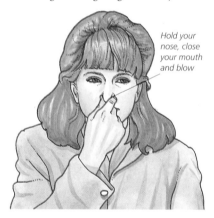

Hold your nose, close your mouth and blow

What you can do
Tell the casualty to swallow with her mouth wide open. If this fails to make the ears "pop", tell the casualty to close her mouth, hold her nose tightly closed and "blow" her nose. If nothing helps, all you can do is reassure the casualty that the pain will go away when the pressure in the middle ear equalises (for example, when the plane lands).

2 Hold a source of heat (such as a covered hot-water bottle) against the affected ear. Let the casualty sit up if lying flat makes the pain worse.

3 Advise the casualty to see her own doctor. If you are worried about the casualty's condition (particularly if a child), call a doctor.

TOOTHACHE

Steady toothache, sometimes made worse by hot or cold food or drinks, is usually due to a decayed tooth. Throbbing toothache indicates an infection; there may be swelling in the painful area, and bad breath. Sometimes what seems to be "toothache" can be caused by conditions such as sinusitis or an ear infection.

TREATMENT

> YOUR AIMS ARE:
> • To relieve pain.
> • To make sure that the casualty sees a dentist.

1 A child may be given the recommended dose of paracetamol syrup; an adult may take two tablets of paracetamol, or his or her own painkillers.

2 Arrange an early appointment with the casualty's dentist. Meanwhile:
• The casualty may plug a cavity with cotton wool soaked in oil of cloves, or hold a small measure of neat spirits in his or her mouth, next to the tooth.
• Give the casualty a covered hot-water bottle to hold to the face.
• Prop the casualty up with pillows if lying down makes the pain worse.

ABDOMINAL PAIN

Pain in the abdomen may be relatively trivial (for example, indigestion) but can indicate very serious disease, such as perforation or obstruction of the intestine.

Obstruction or distension of the intestine causes pain that fluctuates in intensity (colic), often causing the sufferer to "double up in agony" or roll about, and is frequently accompanied by vomiting. Perforation, or leakage into the abdominal cavity, causes intense, steady pain, often very sudden and made worse by any movement.

Mild colic may respond to simple remedies, but serious, persistent pain must receive medical attention.

TREATMENT

> YOUR AIMS ARE:
> • To relieve pain and discomfort.
> • To obtain medical aid if necessary.

1 Make the casualty comfortable, propped up if breathing is difficult. Provide a container in case he or she is sick.

> DO NOT give any medicines or anything to eat or drink.

2 Give the casualty a covered hot-water bottle to place against the abdomen.

IF the pain is severe, or does not ease within 30 minutes, call a doctor.

> **Winding**
> A blow to the upper abdomen may stun a local nerve junction, causing a temporary breathing problem. Sit the casualty down, and loosen clothing at the chest or waist. Recovery should be rapid.

DIARRHOEA AND VOMITING

This is most likely to be due to food poisoning, the consumption of contaminated water or, sometimes, unusual or exotic foods. Diarrhoea may, of course, occur without vomiting, and vice versa.

When both occur together there is an increased risk of dehydration, especially in infants and young children.

See also: Food poisoning, *page 172.*

TREATMENT

YOUR AIM IS:
• To restore lost fluid and salts.

1 Give the casualty plenty of bland fluids to drink, slowly and often.

2 When the appetite returns, give only bland, starchy food for 24 hours.

Suitable drinks
"Isotonic" glucose drinks, and the special replacement fluids available in powder form from chemists, are ideal. Or, add salt (1 teaspoonful per litre) and sugar (4 or 5 teaspoonfuls per litre) to either water or dilute orange juice, which is a useful source of potassium.

HERNIA

A hernia ("rupture") is a protrusion of parts of the contents of the abdomen (often a small loop of intestine) through a weak part of the muscular wall. It may result from heavy exertion or coughing. The swelling may be painless and disappear if the casualty lies down. If it is painful, especially if accompanied by vomiting and abdominal pain, the hernia is said to be "strangulated", and requires urgent medical attention.

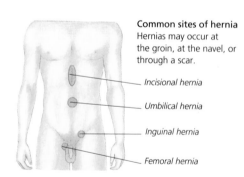

Common sites of hernia
Hernias may occur at the groin, at the navel, or through a scar.

— *Incisional hernia*

— *Umbilical hernia*

— *Inguinal hernia*

— *Femoral hernia*

TREATMENT

YOUR AIM IS:
• To obtain medical attention.

FOR A PAINLESS HERNIA

Reassure the casualty. Without causing unnecessary alarm, advise the casualty to see his or her own doctor as soon as possible. Do not push the swelling in.

FOR A PAINFUL HERNIA

1 Make the casualty comfortable, with bent knees and back well supported.

2 Call a doctor or, if the pain is severe, dial 999 for an ambulance.

DO NOT push the swelling in.

CRAMP

This is a sudden, involuntary, and painful muscle spasm. It commonly happens during sleep, but can also be caused by strenuous exercise, such as running, or by the loss of excessive salt and fluid from the body through profuse sweating. Cramp can often be relieved by stretching and massaging the affected muscle.

See also: Heat exhaustion, page 133.

TREATMENT

YOUR AIM IS:
- To relieve both spasm and pain.

FOR CRAMP IN THE FOOT

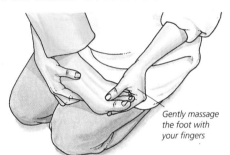

Gently massage the foot with your fingers

Help the casualty to stand with his weight on the front of his foot. When the first spasm has passed, massage the foot.

FOR CRAMP IN THE CALF

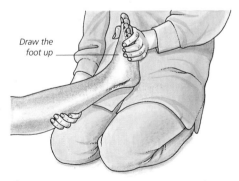

Draw the foot up

Straighten the casualty's knee, and draw her foot firmly and steadily upwards toward the shin. Massage the muscles.

FOR CRAMP IN THE THIGH

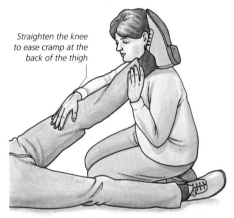

Straighten the knee to ease cramp at the back of the thigh

For cramp in the back of the thigh, straighten the casualty's knee by raising the leg. For cramp in the front of the thigh, bend the knee. In each case, massage the muscle firmly with your fingers.

Stitch

This common condition is caused by overuse of the muscles of the abdominal wall. These muscles contract while we run or walk quickly, to help us retain an upright posture. If they are used excessively and become fatigued, the muscle fibres become deprived of oxygen. The pain of stitch thus feels similar to that of angina (see page 72).

What you can do
The casualty must sit down and rest; the pain will usually ease within a few minutes. No other treatment is required.

HYSTERIA

This is rather a vague term, and is often incorrectly used. True hysteria is a sub-conscious condition, caused by psycho-logical stress, that manifests itself as some physical complaint, such as blindness.

We are more likely, however, to apply the term "hysterical" to someone who is "over-reacting", possibly at the scene of an accident, or on learning that a relative has died, or been killed. People with this "reactionary hysteria" need to be handled firmly and positively.

RECOGNITION

There may be:
- Attention-seeking loss of behavioural control – shouting, screaming, rolling on the ground, or beating the chest – usually made worse by an audience.
- Hyperventilation, possibly extreme, inducing spasm in the wrists and hands.
- Marked tremor or "paralysis"; the casualty is apparently unable to move.

See also: Hyperventilation, *page 62.*

TREATMENT

YOUR AIM IS:
- To help the casualty to calm down and regain self-control.

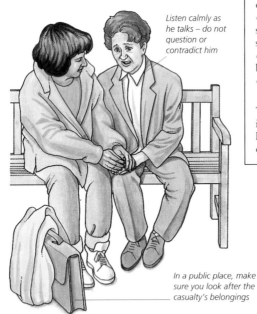

Listen calmly as he talks – do not question or contradict him

In a public place, make sure you look after the casualty's belongings

Panic attack

Some people occasionally display anxiety out of proportion to the stress they are actually experiencing. Signs and symptoms of a panic attack include:
- Nervous overactivity – trembling, sweating, palpitations, and difficulty in swallowing.
- Tension – producing headaches, backache, and pressure in the chest.
- Hyperventilation (*see page 62*).

What you can do
Treat as for hysteria. It is very important that the casualty sees his or her doctor, so that the underlying state of anxiety can be treated.

DO NOT throw water at the casualty's face.

DO NOT slap the casualty's face.

DO NOT use force to restrain him.

1 Escort the casualty to a quiet place, away from onlookers. Be firm and positive; do not over-sympathise.

2 Stay with the casualty quietly until he has recovered. Advise him to consult his doctor.

HICCUPS

These short, repeated, noisy intakes of air are caused by involuntary contractions of the diaphragm, working against a partially closed windpipe. Hiccups do not usually last more than a few minutes; short attacks are simply a nuisance, but if an attack is prolonged it may become worrying, tiring, and painful.

TREATMENT

YOUR AIM IS:
• To temporarily increase carbon dioxide levels in the blood.

1 Try any or all of the following methods:
• Tell the casualty to sit quietly and hold his breath for as long as possible.
• Make him take long drinks from the "wrong" side of a cup or glass.
• Place a paper (*not* plastic) bag over the nose and mouth and get the casualty to re-breathe his expired air for a minute.

IF the hiccups persist for more than a few hours, call a doctor for advice.

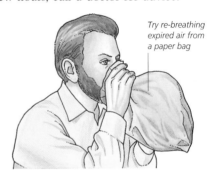
Try re-breathing expired air from a paper bag

ALLERGY

In the same way that the body makes antibodies to combat germs, it may also make antibodies to other substances – pollen, foods, chemicals, drugs – which may be touched, inhaled, or swallowed. This results in an *allergy* – an adverse reaction, caused by a hypersensitivity to some substance that is not generally recognised to be harmful. Allergies generally cause problems in one of three ways, but reactions can be mixed or overlap.
• Respiratory allergies may result in asthma (*see page 163*) or in hay fever.
• Intestinal allergies may produce vomiting, abdominal pain, and diarrhoea (*see page 184*).
• Skin allergies may take the form of "nettle rash" (*urticaria*) or dermatitis. Anaphylactic shock is the name given to a rare, generalised, and dangerous allergic reaction that requires urgent and specialised medical attention.

See also: Anaphylactic shock, *page 71.*

TREATMENT

YOUR AIM IS:
• To recognise the problem and treat any physical symptoms.

1 Treat any symptoms possible – for example, diarrhoea.

2 Advise the casualty to see his or her doctor. Call a doctor if in doubt.

ILLNESS AND OVERSEAS TRAVEL

With the rise in availability of air travel, many people now find themselves at risk from diseases that are not commonly encountered in the United Kingdom. A hot climate brings problems of its own to those unused to it, such as the risks of sunburn and heat exhaustion.

The value of good preparation

When planning any foreign travel, obtain as much information as you can about the health problems of the area to be visited. Many conditions encountered abroad can be avoided by common-sense measures (*see below*), and some can be prevented by vaccination (available from your doctor) before departure.

See also: Bites and stings, *pages 97-102*.
Diarrhoea and vomiting, *page 184*.
The effects of extreme heat, *page 133*.
Rabies, *page 98*.
Sunburn, *page 112*.

COMMON CONDITIONS ENCOUNTERED OVERSEAS

Condition	Cause and features	Prevention
Malaria	The most common disease in the world, malaria affects around 200 million people every year. It is transmitted by mosquito bite and is prevalent in almost all tropical and sub-tropical areas. In the early stages malaria resembles 'flu, with fever and headache.	Wear enveloping clothing, use insect repellent and mosquito nets, and take anti-malarial tablets; these tablets must be started before travel and continued on return. Anyone developing a fever in, or on return from, an infected area should be seen by a doctor.
Prickly heat	This is a highly irritating, prickly red rash caused by inflamed sweat glands that particularly affects areas that are not well-aerated. Sufferers are more than usually liable to heatstroke.	Maintain good personal hygiene, and wear clean, loose clothing made of natural fibres. Sufferers should spend as much time as possible in cool conditions, and should certainly avoid exercise in the heat.
Fungal infections	Conditions such as "athlete's foot" are common in warm climates and can be more than usually painful and incapacitating. These fungal infections commonly affect the groin ("dhobi itch"), between the toes, and the armpits, causing great discomfort.	Maintain good personal hygiene and wear clean, loose clothing made of natural fibres. Use plenty of medicated talcum powder.
Swimmer's ear	Swimmer's ear is an infective inflammation of the external ear canal. It can be very troublesome and difficult to cure.	Wear well-fitting ear plugs and take care to dry the ears thoroughly after swimming.

EMERGENCY CHILDBIRTH

T here are two situations in which you may need to administer first aid to a pregnant woman: miscarriage and childbirth.

Miscarriage is a common but upsetting and possibly dangerous event. It is important that the woman receives medical attention, and that she is treated with sensitivity, both during and after this distressing experience.

Emergency childbirth

Though the newspapers revel in stories of births in unusual circumstances, emergency childbirth is rare. The main thing is not to panic; childbirth is a natural and often lengthy process. There is usually plenty of time during which to get help.

Nevertheless, it is important that, in an emergency, you know what you can and should do, and what you should not do. Remember, too, that women were giving birth long before first aid was taught; the mother, particularly if she has given birth before, may be a valuable source of information. The woman herself may be able to direct operations during delivery.

THE FIRST AIDER SHOULD:

Miscarriage:
• Ensure that the woman receives medical attention as soon as possible.

Childbirth:
• Keep calm. Conceal any anxiety you may feel, and reassure the mother.
• Seek expert help as soon as possible. Male First Aiders may also wish to seek a female chaperone.
• Never try to delay childbirth in any way.

MISCARRIAGE

A miscarriage is the loss of the embryo or foetus at any time before the 28th week of pregnancy. About 20 per cent of all pregnancies end in miscarriage, many women miscarrying without even being aware that they are pregnant.

Some women experience a "threatened miscarriage" with only slight vaginal bleeding. Complete miscarriages carry the danger of severe bleeding and shock. Any woman who is, or appears to be, miscarrying must be seen by a doctor.

Remember that the woman may be frightened and very distressed. Though your efforts may be rejected, try and offer as much help as you can without being intrusive. A woman who suspects that she is miscarrying may be reluctant to confide in a stranger, particularly if that person is a man.

RECOGNITION

There may be:
* Cramp-like pains in her lower abdomen or pelvic area.
* Vaginal bleeding, possibly sudden and profuse.
* Signs of shock.
* Passage of the foetus and other products of conception.

See also: Shock, *page 68.*

TREATMENT

> YOUR AIMS ARE:
> • To reassure and comfort the woman.
> • To obtain medical attention.

1 Reassure the woman. Help her to lie down in a semi-reclining position.

2 Give her a sanitary pad or clean towel.

3 Check and record pulse and breathing rate.

4 Keep any expelled material (out of the woman's sight, if possible) for medical inspection.

IF the bleeding and/or pains are only slight, call a doctor.

IF bleeding and/or pain is severe, dial 999 for an ambulance. Treat the woman for shock.

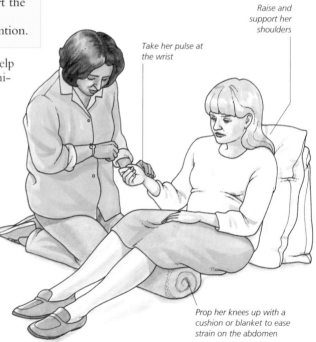

Raise and support her shoulders

Take her pulse at the wrist

Prop her knees up with a cushion or blanket to ease strain on the abdomen

CHILDBIRTH

The majority of births do not threaten the lives of either mother or baby. Nevertheless, a woman who goes into labour unexpectedly may become very anxious, and you must do your best to reassure and calm her. Labour usually lasts several hours, and there is normally plenty of time to arrange transport to hospital, or for the assistance of a midwife or doctor.

Never try to delay a birth in any way. Allow the delivery to proceed without interfering until the baby's head is emerging. Rarely, the baby's position is reversed and it emerges bottom first (a breech delivery). This requires urgent medical attention.

The stages of childbirth

Labour is divided into three stages:
● First stage (often around 12-14 hours) – dilation of the neck of the womb.
● Second stage (up to 2 hours) – descent of the baby from the womb to the vaginal entrance, and delivery.
● Third stage (up to 30 minutes) – delivery of the afterbirth.

THE FIRST STAGE OF LABOUR

In late pregnancy, the womb contracts intermittently, producing fleeting cramp-like pains. The first stage of labour begins when the neck of the womb (*cervix*) opens and begins to dilate.

Possible signs of labour

Regular contractions become established, gradually increasing in intensity and frequency; 10-20 minutes is an average interval. Full dilation of the cervix may take 12-14 hours for a first child, and less for any subsequent pregnancy.

As the neck of the womb dilates, its mucus plug may be expelled as a bloodstained discharge, or "show". The show may be negligible, or quite heavy, and may signal that labour is beginning.

A membranous bag contains a clear fluid (the *amniotic fluid*) that surrounds and cushions the baby in the womb. When the need for protection ends, this bag of "waters" will break, either in a rush or a steady trickle. This may happen early in the first stage, but it may signal the beginning of the second stage (*see overleaf*).

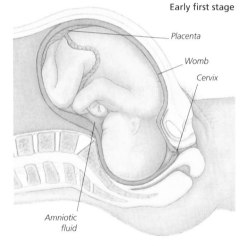

Early first stage

Placenta

Womb

Cervix

Amniotic fluid

WHAT YOU SHOULD DO

1 Summon a midwife or doctor, and an ambulance if necessary.

2 Stay with the mother. Let her walk about, or have a bath, if she wishes.

IF her waters have broken, do not let her have a bath, because there is a risk of infection.

THE SECOND STAGE OF LABOUR

When the cervix is fully dilated, the second stage begins. Without its cushion of fluid, the baby is in close contact with the muscle of the womb. This stimulates stronger, more frequent contractions. The second stage lasts until the baby is delivered, possibly in as little as an hour.

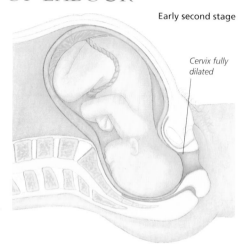

Early second stage

Cervix fully dilated

What happens at the birth

The vagina stretches to allow the baby's head to emerge. Once the head is delivered, the rest of the baby will be pushed out rapidly. The baby will still be attached to the mother by the umbilical cord. It is not necessary for the First Aider to cut the cord. The rest of the cord and placenta are then delivered (*see page 196*).

WHAT YOU WILL NEED

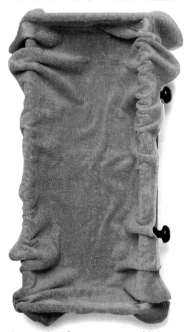

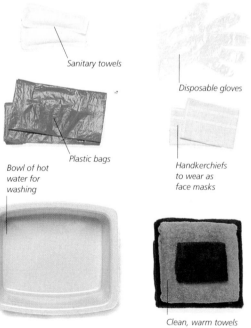

Sanitary towels

Disposable gloves

Plastic bags

Bowl of hot water for washing

Handkerchiefs to wear as face masks

Clean, warm towels

Preparations for an emergency birth

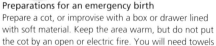

Prepare a cot, or improvise with a box or drawer lined with soft material. Keep the area warm, but do not put the cot by an open or electric fire. You will need towels and absorbent pads (sanitary towels are ideal) to mop up waste; a bag for waste, and a separate one for the afterbirth, which must be preserved for inspection.

PREPARING FOR DELIVERY

The prospective mother is likely to be nervous and excited. Keep calm and reassure her. Arrange a warm, quiet environment and ask for help, preferably from a female relative or neighbour. The father may wish to be present and to help with the delivery; he will generally be of most use at the mother's head, giving comfort and support during contractions.

If the mother is not at home, help her into a half-sitting position on the floor, the seat of a car, or any flat surface. If you are in a public place, ask bystanders to stand with their backs to the mother.

While you should try and keep the number of people present to a minimum, do not exclude anyone the mother wishes to be present.

Preventing infection

When preparing for, and during, the delivery it is extremely important to pay strict attention to hygiene.
- Keep anyone with a cold, sore throat, or septic spots on the hands well away.
- Wear a face mask. You can improvise one from a clean handkerchief or a folded triangular bandage.
- Remove outer clothing and roll up your sleeves. If possible, wear a plastic apron.
- Wash your hands and scrub your nails thoroughly for about five minutes. Wear disposable gloves if available.
- After the delivery, wash your hands thoroughly again.

1 Cover the bed, sofa, or floor with plastic sheeting, towels, or newspaper, and make the woman comfortable.

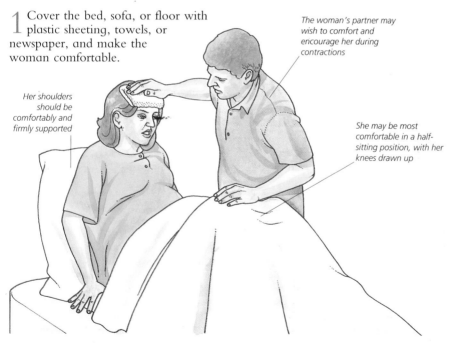

The woman's partner may wish to comfort and encourage her during contractions

Her shoulders should be comfortably and firmly supported

She may be most comfortable in a half-sitting position, with her knees drawn up

2 Ask her to remove any clothing that will interfere with the delivery. During the early second stage, keep her covered with blankets for as long as possible.

3 Put cotton, lint, or sheeting under her buttocks, for warmth and to absorb mess. Place a clean pad over the anus, as involuntary bowel movements may occur.

WHAT YOU SHOULD DO

1 Ensure that an ambulance is on its way. As well as giving your exact location, tell the control the expected delivery date, and the name of the hospital, if any, into which the mother is booked.

2 Tell the mother to grasp her knees or the back of her thighs. This will help her push with the contractions, which by now may be coming every 2-3 minutes.

> DO NOT give the mother anything to eat or drink. If she is thirsty, moisten her lips with water.

IF there is soiling, clean the area from front to back to protect against infection.

3 Inspect the vaginal area. When the *perineum* (between the vagina and the anus) bulges, the baby's head should become visible. Support it as it emerges.

Tell her to bend her head forwards, hold her breath and push down during contractions

4 When the widest part, or crown, of the head is through, tell the mother to stop pushing and pant during the contraction. This will enable you to swiftly examine the head.

> DO NOT pull the baby's head.

Keep supporting the baby's head during and between contractions

5 Check that there is no membrane covering the baby's face. If there is, tear it away.

6 Check that the umbilical cord is not around the baby's neck. If it is, pull it over the baby's head.

7 The baby's head will turn to face to the side. Allow this to happen naturally while supporting the head.

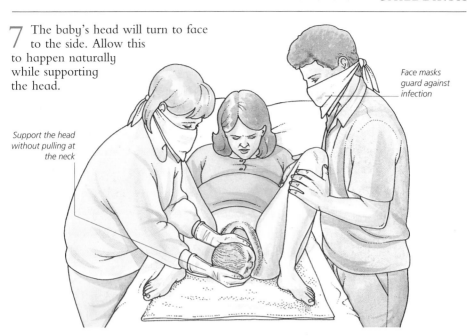

Face masks guard against infection

Support the head without pulling at the neck

8 Continuing support, lower the baby's head until the uppermost shoulder appears at the birth canal.

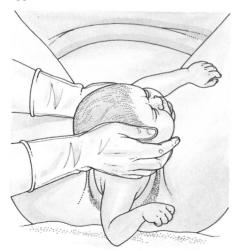

9 Once the first shoulder is clear, lift the head upwards towards the mother's abdomen to free the second shoulder from the birth canal; the rest of the baby will be expelled rapidly.

DO NOT pull at the shoulders.

10 Lift the baby away from the birth canal. Newborn babies are very slippery, and need to be handled carefully. Gently lay the baby on the mother.

DO NOT pull on or cut the umbilical cord (*see overleaf*).

11 Clean out the baby's mouth with a swab. The baby should start to cry; if it does not respond, carry out the ABC of resuscitation (*see page 36*).

DO NOT smack the baby.

12 Wrap the baby and put it in the mother's arms while you attend to the afterbirth (*see overleaf*). Make sure the baby is lying on its side with the head low, so that fluid or mucus can drain from the nose and mouth.

THE THIRD STAGE OF LABOUR

During the third stage, mild contractions continue in order to expel the afterbirth (the *placenta* and cord). This normally takes 10-30 minutes, and there is usually some bleeding. The womb should then contract, closing down the site of the placental attachment and stopping the bleeding. If this mechanism fails, a *post-partum* (after-delivery) haemorrhage may occur; bleeding may be extensive, causing shock to develop (*see page 68*). The cord can safely be left uncut until help arrives, or until mother and baby reach hospital. It may pulsate for a few minutes.

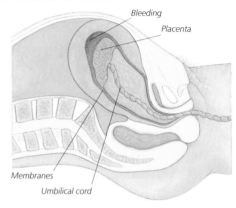

Bleeding

Placenta

Membranes

Umbilical cord

WHAT YOU SHOULD DO

1 Wait and watch until the afterbirth is delivered naturally. Encourage the mother during contractions.

Make sure the woman is comfortable

> DO NOT pull on the cord.
>
> DO NOT cut the cord.

Massaging the woman's abdomen will help the womb to contract and harden, and should stop the bleeding

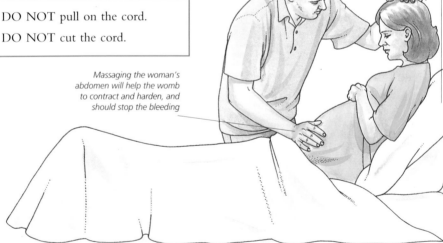

2 Keep the afterbirth intact, preferably in a polythene bag, as it must be examined when the mother reaches hospital. Even a small piece left inside can cause dangerous complications.

3 Clean the mother and lay a sanitary pad or clean towel over her vagina.

4 A small amount of bleeding is normal. Severe bleeding is rare, but manage-able. Keep calm. Gently massage the mother's abdomen just below the navel. Keep up the massage until help arrives.

IF bleeding is severe, treat for shock. Ensure an ambulance is on its way.

DRESSINGS AND BANDAGES

Applying dressings and bandages is an important part of good first aid practice. Wounds usually require a dressing, and almost all injuries will benefit from the support that bandages can give.

How dressings and bandages are used

Dressings can be used to control bleeding, and to cover a wound, protecting it and thereby reducing the risk of infection. Bandages are used to hold dressings in place and to give support to injuries. They may also be used to restrict movement, and to secure splints and cold compresses in place.

What you will find in this chapter

This chapter shows you the materials you need to equip a useful first aid kit, and how to use these materials properly. A practical first aid course will increase your proficiency. The dressing and/or bandage you choose, and the technique for applying it, will vary according to the materials available to you, and the type of injury sustained. More detailed information may be found on the pages dealing with specific injuries.

DRESSINGS ARE USED TO:
- Control bleeding.
- Protect the wound and prevent infection.

BANDAGES ARE USED TO:
- Maintain direct pressure over a dressing.
- Hold dressings and splints in place.
- Limit swelling.
- Provide support to a limb or joint.
- Restrict movement.

CONTENTS

FIRST AID MATERIALS

First aid kits should be kept in your home, your car, and in the workplace. A workplace kit must be readily accessible, and must contain certain items, depending on the nature of the business. The materials in a standard first aid kit make a useful basic kit for the home. You may want to add extra dressings and bandages, adhesive strapping, cotton wool, scissors, tweezers, and disposable gloves. Keep first aid kits in a dry atmosphere (bathrooms are often damp). Check and replenish your kit regularly, so that you always have items you need to hand.

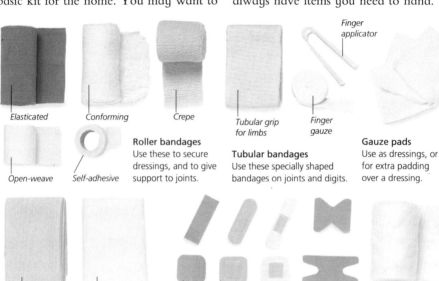

Finger applicator

Elasticated

Conforming

Crepe

Tubular grip for limbs

Finger gauze

Open-weave

Self-adhesive

Roller bandages
Use these to secure dressings, and to give support to joints.

Tubular bandages
Use these specially shaped bandages on joints and digits.

Gauze pads
Use as dressings, or for extra padding over a dressing.

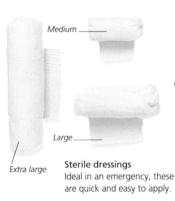

Cloth

Paper

Fabric   Waterproof   Clear   Heel and finger

Cotton wool

Triangular bandages
Made of cloth or strong paper, these can be used as bandages and slings.

Adhesive dressings
Use for minor wounds. The waterproof types are the best choice for wounds on the hands.

Cotton wool
Never place this on a wound; use it as an absorbent outer layer, or as padding.

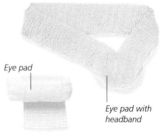

Medium

Eye pad

Large

Extra large

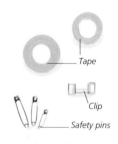

Eye pad with headband

Tape

Clip

Safety pins

Sterile dressings
Ideal in an emergency, these are quick and easy to apply.

Sterile eye pads
Any injury to the eye needs the protection of a sterile covering.

Pins, clips and tape
Use these for securing bandages or dressings.

Basic materials for a first aid kit:
- 10 *adhesive dressings (plasters).*
- 3 *medium-sized sterile dressings.*
- 1 *large sterile dressing.*
- 1 *extra-large sterile dressing.*
- 1 *sterile eye pad.*
- 2 *triangular bandages.*
- 2 *crepe roller bandages.*
- 6 *safety pins.*

Useful additions to first aid kits for camping trips or outdoor activities:
- *A torch.*
- *A whistle.*
- *Blankets.*
- *Extra triangular bandages.*
- *Material for improvised splints.*
- *Extra cotton wool for padding.*
- *A polythene "survival bag".*

Plastic gloves will do in an emergency, though the more robust surgical types are preferable

Disposable gloves
Wear gloves when dressing wounds or disposing of any waste materials.

Notepad and pencil
Keep these handy to record casualties' details, and your observations during treatment.

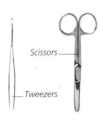

Scissors

Tweezers

Scissors and tweezers
Kept in the kit, these will always be to hand.

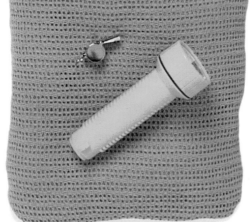

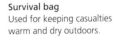

Wound cleansing wipes
These clean the skin around small wounds.

Blanket, torch, and whistle
Add these to outdoor or camping first aid kits. Always keep a torch in your car.

Survival bag
Used for keeping casualties warm and dry outdoors.

DRESSINGS

Although dressings may stick to a wound, their benefits outweigh any discomfort caused on removal. They cover the wound, protect against germs, and help the blood-clotting process. Use a purpose-made, pre-packed sterile dressing whenever possible. If none is available, use any clean, non-fluffy material, such as a triangular bandage or handkerchief, to improvise a dressing. Do not use fluffy materials, which may stick to, and contaminate, the wound.

General rules for applying dressings

• The dressing pad should always extend well beyond a wound's edges.
• Place dressings directly on a wound. Do not slide them on from the side, and replace any that slip from place.
• If bleeding strikes through a dressing, do not remove it; instead, apply another dressing over the top.
• If there is only one sterile dressing, use this to cover the wound, and use other clean materials as top-dressings.

To minimise the risk of introducing germs from your breath or fingers to an open wound:

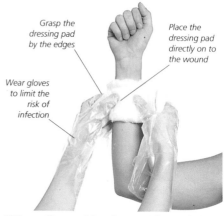

Grasp the dressing pad by the edges

Place the dressing pad directly on to the wound

Wear gloves to limit the risk of infection

• Wear disposable gloves, if available.
• Where possible, wash your hands thoroughly before dressing a wound.
• Avoid touching the wound, or any part of the dressing that will come into contact with the wound.
• Try not to talk, sneeze, or cough over a wound.

Preventing cross-infection

To avoid picking up infection from the casualty, cover cuts and grazes on your hands with waterproof dressings, and wear disposable gloves whenever possible.

Dressing wounds when gloves are unavailable
• Ask the casualty to dress his or her own wound under your supervision.
• Enclose your hands in plastic bags.
• Dress the wound, but wash your hands very thoroughly afterwards.

Dealing with waste
• Mop up blood and body fluid spills as soon as possible (a solution of of 1 part bleach to 10 parts water is recommended).

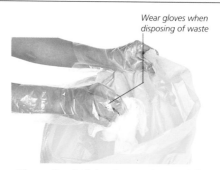

Wear gloves when disposing of waste

• Place all soiled dressings and materials, including gloves, in a plastic bag. Seal the bag and destroy it by incineration.
• Put sharp items in containers for disposal.

STERILE DRESSINGS

Also known as "ambulance dressings", these consist of a dressing pad with a bandage attached. The dressing pad is made up of a piece of gauze or lint backed by a layer of cotton wool padding. Sterile dressings are sold in single units in a variety of sizes, and are sealed in protective wrappings. If the seal on a sterile dressing is broken, the dressing is no longer sterile.

METHOD

1 Remove the wrapping, and find the loose end of the bandage and unwind it. Unfold the sterile pad, being careful not to touch it as you do so.

> DO NOT bandage so tightly that the circulation is impeded.

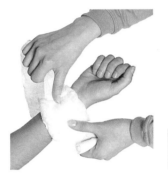 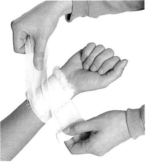 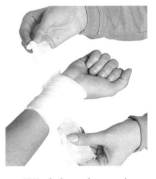

2 Holding the bandage on either side of the pad, place the pad directly on to the wound.

3 Wind the shorter end of the bandage once around the limb and dressing to secure the pad.

4 Wind the other end above and below the loose short end, until the whole pad is covered.

IF the dressing slips from place, remove it and apply a new dressing.

5 Secure the bandage by tying the ends in a reef knot (*see page 212*). Tie the knot over the pad to exert firm pressure over the wound.

IF bleeding strikes through the dressing, do not remove it. Apply another dressing over the top.

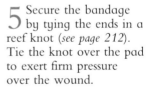

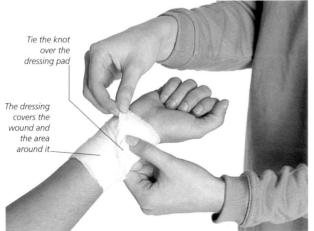

Tie the knot over the dressing pad

The dressing covers the wound and the area around it

6 Check the circulation (*see page 205*).

GAUZE DRESSINGS

If a sterile dressing is not available, gauze pads may be used. These are made from layers of gauze that form a soft, pliable covering for wounds. Cover the gauze with pads of cotton wool to absorb blood or discharge. Use adhesive strapping to secure the dressing, or a roller bandage if pressure is required. If using strapping, do not completely encircle a limb or digit, as this can impede the circulation. Some people's skin reacts to the adhesive used on strapping, so ask before using it.

METHOD

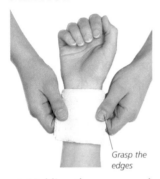
Grasp the edges

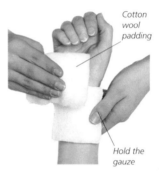
Cotton wool padding

Hold the gauze

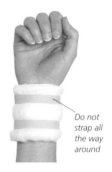
Do not strap all the way around

1 Holding the gauze pad by the edges, place it directly on to the wound.

2 Add a layer of cotton wool padding on top of the gauze.

3 Secure with adhesive strapping, or a roller bandage (see page 207).

ADHESIVE DRESSINGS

Commonly known as "plasters", these are useful for small wounds. They consist of a gauze or cellulose pad attached to an adhesive backing. They come in various sizes, usually as individually wrapped sterile units. Specially shaped plasters are available for fingertips, heels, and elbows. Food handlers are required to wear waterproof plasters, preferably coloured, on cuts and grazes on their hands.

METHOD

1 Remove the wrapping and hold the dressing, pad-side down, by the protective strips.

2 Peel back, but do not remove, the protective strips. Without touching the dressing pad, place it directly on to the wound.

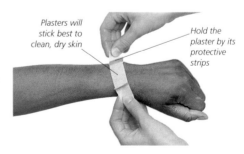
Plasters will stick best to clean, dry skin

Hold the plaster by its protective strips

3 Carefully pull away the protective strips. Press the ends and edges down.

COLD COMPRESSES

Cooling an injury such as a bruise or sprain can help reduce swelling and pain. You can place the injured part directly under cold running water, or in a bowl of cold water. When injuries are on an awkward part of the body, such as the head or chest, or when they need prolonged cooling, use a cold compress. This can be a pad soaked in very cold water, or an ice bag wrapped in cloth. A bag of frozen vegetables, particularly peas, is an excellent alternative to ice cubes.

APPLYING AN ICEPACK

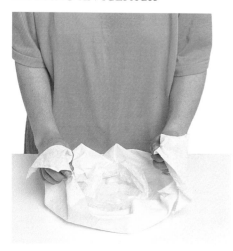

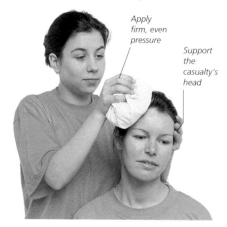

Apply firm, even pressure

Support the casualty's head

1 Fill a plastic bag half to two-thirds full with small ice cubes or, preferably, crushed ice. Knot the top of the bag, and wrap it in a piece of cloth, such as a tea-towel or triangular bandage.

2 Place the icepack over the injury. You may use a roller bandage (*see page 207*) to hold it firmly in position.

3 Continue to cool the injury for 20 minutes, replacing the ice in the pack as necessary.

APPLYING A COLD PAD

1 Soak a flannel or towel in very cold water. Wring it out so that it remains cold and damp, and place it on the injury and the surrounding area.

2 Re-soak the pad in cold water every 5 minutes to keep it cold. Cool the injured part for at least 20 minutes.

IF necessary, you may use a roller bandage (*see page 207*) to keep the cold pad firmly in place.

Wring the pad only so that it is not dripping wet

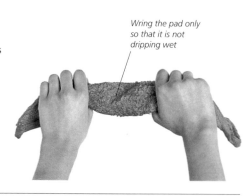

BANDAGES

Bandages have a number of purposes; they are used to hold dressings in place, to control bleeding, to support and immobilise injuries, and to reduce swelling. There are three main types:
• Triangular bandages, which are usually made of cloth; they are used as slings, and also to secure dressings and to immobilise injured limbs.
• Roller bandages, which secure dressings, and can give support to limbs.
• Tubular bandages, which can secure dressings on digits, or support joints.

In an emergency, bandages can be improvised from pieces of cloth, or from items of clothing (*see page 216*).

GENERAL RULES FOR BANDAGING

Before applying bandages:
• Explain to the casualty what you are going to do, and keep reassuring him.

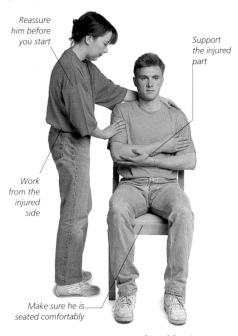

Reassure him before you start

Support the injured part

Work from the injured side

Make sure he is seated comfortably

When applying bandages:
• If the casualty is lying down, pass bandages under the body's natural hollows at the ankles, knees, small of back, and neck. Slide bandages towards the injured area by easing them back and forth.

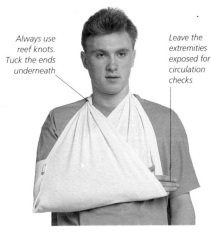

Always use reef knots. Tuck the ends underneath

Leave the extremities exposed for circulation checks

• Make the casualty comfortable, in a sitting or lying position, if possible.
• Keep the injured part supported. The casualty may be able to do this for you.
• Always work in front of the casualty, and from the injured side where possible.

• Apply bandages firmly enough to control any bleeding and hold a dressing in place, but not so tightly as to impede the circulation (*see opposite*).
• Leave fingers and toes on a bandaged limb exposed, if possible, so that you can check the circulation afterwards.
• Ensure knots do not hurt the casualty: use reef knots, tucking the ends underneath, and do not knot over bony areas.

When bandaging to immobilise a limb:

● Make sure there is padding between the limb and body, or between the legs, especially around the joints. Use towels, cotton wool, or folded clothing, and insert the padding before tying the bandages.
● Tie knots at the front of the body on the uninjured side, avoiding bony areas. If both sides of the body are injured, tie the knots in the middle of the body.

After applying bandages:

● Check the circulation in a bandaged limb every 10 minutes (*see below*). Ensure that the blood flow is not impeded.

Bandaging to immobilise a leg

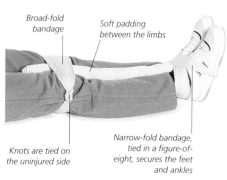

Broad-fold bandage

Soft padding between the limbs

Knots are tied on the uninjured side

Narrow-fold bandage, tied in a figure-of-eight, secures the feet and ankles

CHECKING THE CIRCULATION

You must check the circulation in a hand or foot immediately after bandaging a limb, and again every 10 minutes until medical aid is obtained.

Re-checking the circulation is important because limbs swell following an injury, and a bandage applied immediately after an injury occurred can quickly become too tight and impede the circulation.

RECOGNITION OF IMPAIRED CIRCULATION

There may be:

● Pale, cold skin on the hand or foot.
● Later, a dusky grey/blue appearance to the skin.
● Tingling or numbness.
● Inability to move the affected part.

CHECKING FOR IMPAIRED CIRCULATION

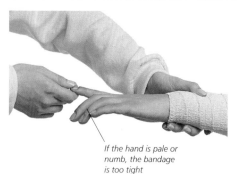

If the hand is pale or numb, the bandage is too tight

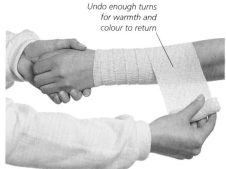

Undo enough turns for warmth and colour to return

1 Press one of the nails, or the skin of the hand or foot, until it is pale. On releasing the pressure, the colour should quickly return. If the nail-bed or skin remains pale, the bandage is too tight.

2 Loosen tight bandages by unrolling just enough turns for warmth and colour to return to the extremity. The casualty may feel a tingling sensation. Reapply the bandage as necessary.

ROLLER BANDAGES

These are used to secure dressings, to apply pressure to control bleeding, and to give support to sprains or strains. They are made of cotton, gauze, or linen, and are applied in spiral turns. Roller bandages may be secured with pins, clips, or tape, but can also be tied off (*see below*).

Types of roller bandage

There are three principal types:
• Open-weave bandages, which are used to hold light dressings in place. Because of their loose weave, they allow good ventilation, but cannot be used to exert pressure on the wound, or to give support to joints.
• Conforming bandages, which are used to secure dressings and to provide light support to injuries.

• Crepe bandages, which are used to give firm support to joints.

Sizes of roller bandage

Before applying a roller bandage, make sure it is tightly rolled and of a suitable width. Remember that it is better for a bandage to be too wide than too narrow; use the chart below to help you choose the right size.

Choosing the best size

Different parts of the body require different widths of roller bandage. These are the recommended sizes for an adult:

Finger	2.5cm (1in)
Hand	5cm (2in)
Arm	7.5-10cm (3-4in)
Leg	10-15cm (4-6in)

Securing roller bandages

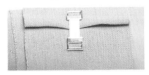

Bandage clips
These are sometimes supplied with elasticated and crepe roller bandages.

Adhesive tape
The ends of bandages can be stuck down with small strips of adhesive strapping.

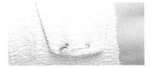

Safety pins
These are often readily available, and can secure all types of roller bandage.

Tying off roller bandages

1 After applying a roller bandage (*see opposite*), leave enough of the end free to allow it to pass around the limb once and tie a knot.

2 Cut down the centre of the loose end, and tie a knot at the bottom of the split.

3 Pass the ends once around the limb, one in each direction, and tie them in a reef knot (*see page 212*).

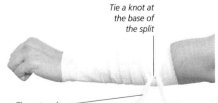

Tie a knot at the base of the split

The cut ends are passed around the limb

APPLYING A ROLLER BANDAGE

Follow these general rules when applying roller bandages:

• When the bandage is partly unrolled, the roll is called the "head", and the unrolled part, the "tail". Keep the head uppermost when bandaging.

• Position yourself in front of the injury.

• Support the injured part in the position it will remain in after bandaging.

• To begin bandaging, place the tail to the limb. Make two straight turns with the head to anchor the bandage.

• Make spiral turns with the bandage, working from the inner side outwards, and from below the injury upwards.

• Check the circulation (*see page 205*) beyond a bandage, especially when using conforming and crepe bandages; these mould to the shape of the limb, and may become tighter if the limb swells.

METHOD

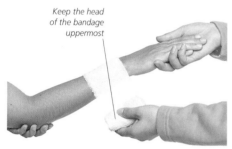

Keep the head of the bandage uppermost

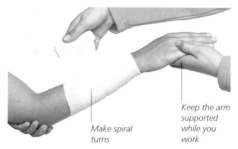

Keep the arm supported while you work

Make spiral turns

1 Place the tail of the bandage below the injury and, working from the inside of the limb outwards, make two straight turns with the bandage head.

2 Make a series of spiral turns, working up the limb. Allow each successive turn to cover between a half and two-thirds of the previous layer.

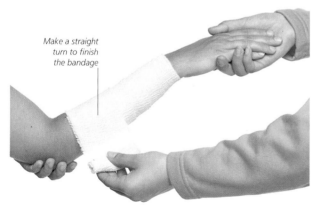

Make a straight turn to finish the bandage

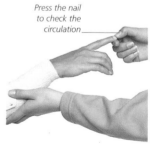

Press the nail to check the circulation

3 Finish off with one straight turn, and secure the end (*see opposite*).

IF the bandage is too short, apply another one in the same way to extend it.

4 Check the circulation (*see page 205*) in the injured limb. If the bandage is too tight, partially undo it, and reapply it more loosely.

ELBOW AND KNEE BANDAGE

Roller bandages can be used at these joints to hold dressings in place, or to support soft tissue injuries such as strains or sprains. Always make sure that your bandaging extends sufficiently far on either side to exert even pressure. The method below, for bandaging an elbow, can also be used for a knee.

METHOD

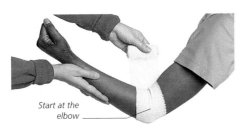

Start at the elbow

1 Support the injured arm in a semi-flexed position. If this is not possible, support the arm in the position most comfortable for the casualty.

2 Place the tail of the bandage on the inside of the elbow, and pass the bandage around the elbow 1½ times, so that the elbow joint is covered.

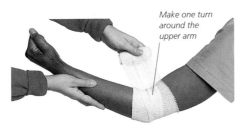

Make one turn around the upper arm

3 Take the head of the bandage above the elbow to the upper arm, and make one turn, covering half of the bandage from the first turn.

4 Take the head of the bandage under the elbow to just below the joint, and make one turn around the lower arm, covering half of the first straight turn.

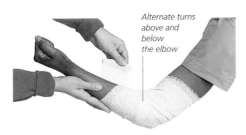

Alternate turns above and below the elbow

5 Continue to alternate these turns, steadily extending the bandaging by covering only between half and two-thirds of the previous layer each time.

DO NOT bandage so tightly that the circulation is impeded.

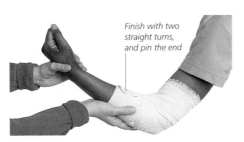

Finish with two straight turns, and pin the end

6 Make two straight turns to finish off, and secure the end (*see page 206*).

7 Check and re-check the circulation (*see page 205*). This is particularly important with this type of bandaging.

IF the bandage is too tight, undo it until the blood supply to the hand returns, then re-bandage more loosely.

HAND AND FOOT BANDAGE

A roller bandage may be used to hold dressings in place on the hand or foot, or to provide support to wrists or ankles that have been sprained or strained. Support bandaging should extend well beyond the joint to provide pressure over the injured area. The method below, for bandaging a hand, can also be used for a foot.

METHOD

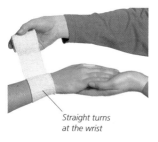

Keep the arm supported

Straight turns at the wrist

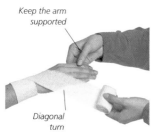

Diagonal turn

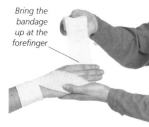

Bring the bandage up at the forefinger

1 Support the casualty's arm. Place the tail of the bandage on the inside of the wrist, at the base of the thumb, and make two straight turns.

2 Take the bandage diagonally across the back of the casualty's hand, so that the edge meets the base of the nail of the little finger.

3 Take the bandage under and around the fingers, and up at the forefinger (so that the edge is at the base of the nail of the forefinger).

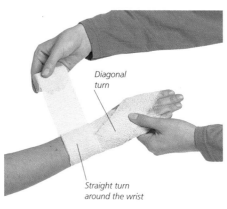

Diagonal turn

Straight turn around the wrist

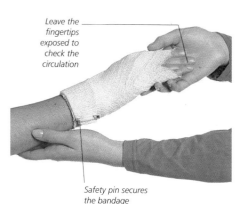

Leave the fingertips exposed to check the circulation

Safety pin secures the bandage

4 Take the bandage diagonally across the back of the hand to the wrist, and then around the wrist and up.

5 Repeat the sequence of turns, covering three-quarters of the bandage from the previous turn each time. Work towards the wrist, leaving the thumb free.

6 When the whole hand is covered, make two straight turns at the wrist and secure the bandage (see page 206).

7 Check the circulation (see page 205) in the hand. If the bandage is too tight, undo it as much as is necessary, and reapply it more loosely.

TUBULAR GAUZE

This is a tubular bandage, made of a roll of seamless gauze. It is useful for holding light dressings in place on a finger or toe, though it cannot exert enough pressure to control bleeding. A special applicator is provided with the roll when it is bought. Tubular gauze bandages are most easily secured with adhesive strapping.

METHOD

1 Cut a piece of tubular gauze 2½ times the length of the finger to be bandaged. Push the whole length on to the applicator. Gently slide the applicator over the injured finger.

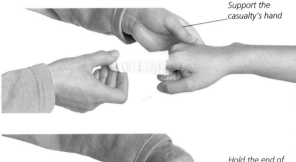

Support the casualty's hand

2 Holding the end of the gauze down at the base of the finger, pull the applicator away until the finger is covered with a layer of gauze, and another remains on the applicator. Twist the applicator twice, holding it slightly away from the fingertip to avoid pinching.

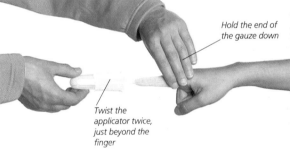

Hold the end of the gauze down

Twist the applicator twice, just beyond the finger

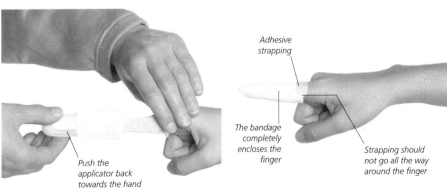

Push the applicator back towards the hand

Adhesive strapping

The bandage completely encloses the finger

Strapping should not go all the way around the finger

3 Gently push the applicator back over the finger until it is covered with the second layer of gauze. Remove the applicator.

4 Secure the bandage with adhesive strapping. Do not completely encircle the finger with strapping, as this may impede the circulation.

TRIANGULAR BANDAGES

These are sold singly in sterile packs, or can be made by cutting or folding a square metre of sturdy fabric (such as linen or calico) diagonally in half. They can be used:

• Straight from a pack and folded into a pad as an improvised sterile dressing pad.

• Open, as slings, or to secure a hand, foot, or scalp dressing.

• Folded into broad-fold bandages (*see below left*), to support and immobilise limbs, and to secure splints and bulky dressings.

• Folded into narrow-fold bandages (*see below right*), to immobilise feet and ankles, and secure dressings to limbs.

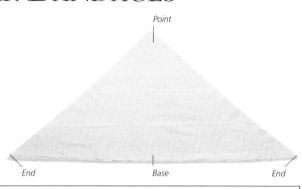

Point

End   Base   End

Storing a triangular bandage

Store triangular bandages in their packs, or this way so that, in an emergency, they are either ready-folded for use, or can simply be shaken open.

1 Start with a narrow-fold bandage (*see below*). Bring the two ends of the bandage into the centre.

2 Keep folding the ends into the centre until a convenient size is reached. Keep in a dry place.

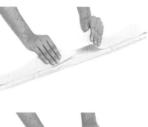

MAKING A BROAD-FOLD BANDAGE

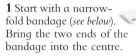

1 Fold a triangular bandage horizontally so that the point touches the base.

2 Fold the bandage in half again. This completes the bandage.

MAKING A NARROW-FOLD BANDAGE

1 Fold a triangular bandage into a broad-fold bandage (*see left*).

2 Fold the bandage in half again. This completes the bandage.

REEF KNOTS

Always use reef knots when tying bandages. They lie flat, are more comfortable for the casualty, will not slip, and are easy to untie. Once the knot is tied, tuck the ends underneath it so that the knot does not press into the casualty's flesh.

TYING A REEF KNOT

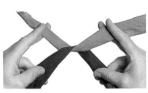

1 Pass the left end over the right, and under.

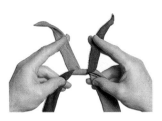

2 Bring both ends up again.

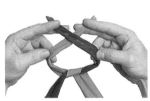

3 Pass the right end over the left, and under.

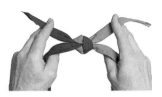

4 Pull the ends firmly. This tightens and completes the knot.

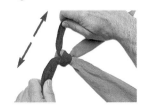

5 *To untie a reef knot:* Pull one end and one piece of bandage apart.

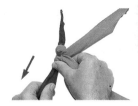

6 Holding the knot, pull the end straight through it and out.

HAND AND FOOT BANDAGE

A triangular bandage may be used to secure a dressing on a hand or foot, though this type of bandage cannot exert enough pressure to control bleeding. The method shown below, for a hand, can also be used for a foot.

METHOD

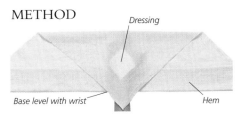

Dressing

Base level with wrist

Hem

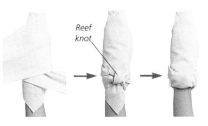

Reef knot

1 Fold a hem along the base of the bandage. Place the casualty's hand, dressing uppermost, on the bandage, and bring the point over to the wrist.

2 Pass the two ends around the wrist, cross them, and tie off. Pull the point to tighten the bandage, bring it up over the knot, and tuck it in underneath.

SCALP BANDAGE

An unfolded triangular bandage may be used to hold a light dressing in place on the scalp, though it cannot exert enough pressure to control bleeding. If possible, sit the casualty down; this makes it easier to apply the bandage.

METHOD

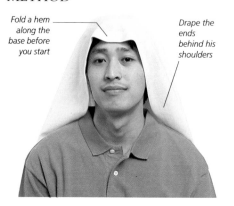

Fold a hem along the base before you start

Drape the ends behind his shoulders

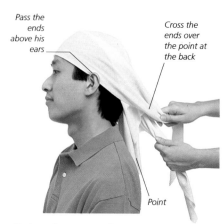

Pass the ends above his ears

Cross the ends over the point at the back

Point

1 Centre the base of the bandage on the casualty's forehead, so that it lies just above the eyebrows. Let the point hang down at the back of the head.

2 Bring the two ends around the head, just above the ears, to the back. Cross the two ends over the point of the bandage at the nape of the neck.

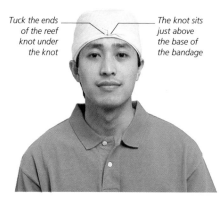

Tuck the ends of the reef knot under the knot

The knot sits just above the base of the bandage

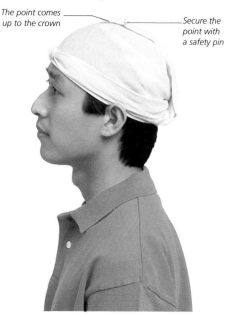

The point comes up to the crown

Secure the point with a safety pin

3 Bring the two ends around to the front and tie off at the centre of the forehead, using a reef knot (*see opposite*).

4 Steadying the casualty's head, draw the point down to tighten the bandage, then take it up to the crown of the head, and secure with a safety pin.

213

SLINGS

Slings can be made from triangular bandages, or any square metre of strong cloth, cut or folded diagonally. There are two different types of slings:
- Arm slings are used to support injured arms or wrists, or to take the weight of the arm off a dislocated shoulder.
- Elevation slings are used to support the arm in cases of collar bone or shoulder injuries. In addition, because the hand is raised, elevation slings should be used for hand injuries, as they help to control bleeding and reduce swelling.

Apply slings from the casualty's injured side. The casualty should be seated, and supporting the injured arm, if possible.

APPLYING AN ARM SLING

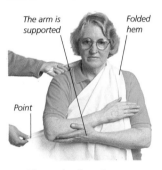

The arm is supported

Folded hem

Point

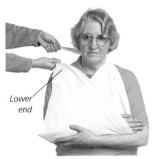

Lower end

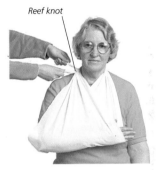

Reef knot

1 Place the bandage between the arm and the chest. Pull one end up around the back of the neck to the injured side.

2 Bring the lower end of the bandage up over the casualty's forearm to meet the other end at the shoulder.

3 Tie a reef knot (*see page 212*) at the hollow over the collar bone on the injured side, and tuck the ends underneath.

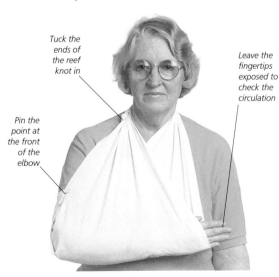

Tuck the ends of the reef knot in

Pin the point at the front of the elbow

Leave the fingertips exposed to check the circulation

4 To secure the point, bring it in front of the elbow. Tuck any loose bandage underneath it, and fasten it above the elbow with a safety pin.

IF you do not have a pin, twist the point round until the sling fits the elbow snugly. Tuck the point into the sling at the front of the arm.

5 Check the circulation (*see page 205*) in the injured part. If the circulation is impeded, undo the sling and loosen any underlying bandages.

APPLYING AN ELEVATION SLING

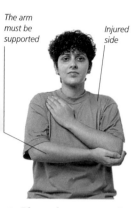

The arm must be supported

Injured side

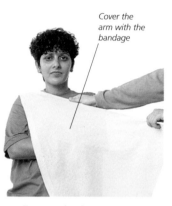

Cover the arm with the bandage

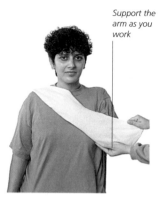

Support the arm as you work

1 Place the arm on the affected side across the chest, with the fingertips touching the opposite shoulder.

2 Drape the bandage over the casualty's arm, with one end over the shoulder, and the point well beyond the elbow on the injured side.

3 Ask the casualty to release her arm. Supporting the arm, tuck the base under her forearm and behind her elbow.

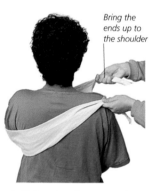

Bring the ends up to the shoulder

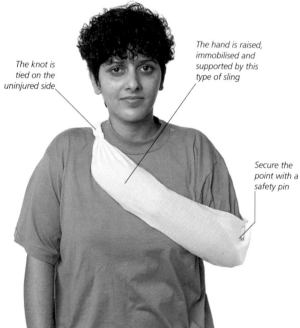

The knot is tied on the uninjured side

The hand is raised, immobilised and supported by this type of sling

Secure the point with a safety pin

4 Bring the lower end up diagonally across her back to meet the other end at the shoulder.

5 Tie a reef knot (see page 212) in the hollow above the casualty's collar bone. Tuck the ends under the knot.

6 Fold the point forward, tucking any loose bandage underneath. Fasten it with a safety pin.

IF you do not have a pin, twist the point and tuck it in at the front of the arm.

IF the casualty's hand feels numb, undo the sling and loosen any bandages.

IMPROVISED SLINGS

You can improvise a sling with a square of cloth. Make sure it is sturdy enough and large enough to support the arm.

You can also improvise slings from pieces of your clothing, or adjust the casualty's clothes to support an injured upper limb.

TO IMPROVISE A SLING

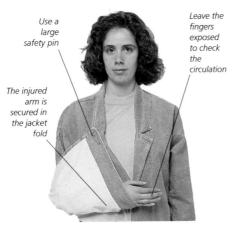

Use a large safety pin

Leave the fingers exposed to check the circulation

The injured arm is secured in the jacket fold

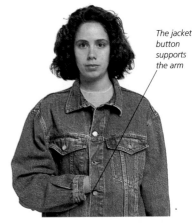

The jacket button supports the arm

• If the casualty is wearing a jacket, undo it, and turn the hem of the jacket up and over the injured arm, and pin it to the jacket breast.

• If the casualty is wearing a button-up coat, jacket or waistcoat, you can undo a button and place the hand of the injured arm inside the fastening.

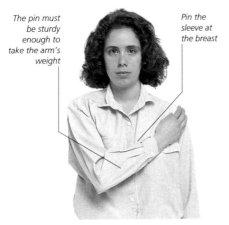

The pin must be sturdy enough to take the arm's weight

Pin the sleeve at the breast

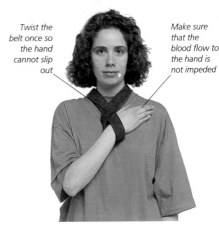

Twist the belt once so the hand cannot slip out

Make sure that the blood flow to the hand is not impeded

• Pin the casualty's sleeve to the opposite breast of her shirt or jacket. For an improvised elevation sling, pin the sleeve further up at the shoulder.

• You can use a belt, a tie, or a pair of braces or tights to make a "collar-and-cuff" support. Do not use this method if you suspect that the forearm is broken.

216

HANDLING AND TRANSPORT

M oving a casualty carries with it the very real risk that you may aggravate his or her injury or condition. Therefore, never move a casualty unless he or she is in immediate danger, or must be moved to shelter while you are waiting for medical help to arrive. Nor must you ever endanger your own safety to move a casualty.

What you will find in this chapter

This chapter shows you the recommended techniques for lifting or dragging a casualty away from danger. There is also advice on the different types of stretcher, and how to use them when transport is necessary.

Comprehensive instruction can only be given in a practical first aid training course. The regular, uniformed, or professional First Aider may also consult ambulance aid training manuals for further information on handling and transport.

HANDLING AND TRANSPORT RULES:

• Do not move a casualty unless absolutely necessary. Do not endanger your own safety.

• Always explain to a casualty what you are doing, so that he or she can co-operate, if possible.

• Never move a casualty alone if help is available. Make sure helpers understand what they are to do, so that they can co-operate fully.

• When several people are moving a casualty, one person only gives verbal commands.

• To protect yourself from back injury when lifting or carrying a casualty, always use the correct lifting technique.

CONTENTS

MANUAL LIFTS AND CARRIES

The method you choose to remove a casualty from immediate danger will depend on the situation, the casualty's condition, and whether there is anyone available to help (*see below*).

In less urgent circumstances – for example, to get a casualty to shelter while waiting for specialist help and equipment to arrive – a more planned approach to transport, using stretchers, can be made.

- Never attempt to move a seriously ill or injured person unless there is an immediate threat to life.
- Never presume that a casualty can sit or stand without support.
- Never move a casualty on your own when help is available.
- Assess the lifting capabilities of your helpers in relation to the task.
- Make sure that everyone involved understands what is to be done.

LIFTS AND CARRIES FOR ONE AND TWO FIRST AIDERS

Condition of casualty	One First Aider	Two First Aiders
Conscious, able to walk	Human crutch	Human crutch
Conscious, unable to walk	Pick-a-back (light-weight casualties only) Drag method (may aggravate head or neck injuries)	Two-handed seat Fore-and-aft carry (not for casualties with arm injuries)
Unconscious	Cradle method (light-weight casualties only) Drag method (see above)	Fore-and-aft carry (see above)

How to lift correctly

Lifting and lowering should not harm the casualty or yourself. Always use your strongest muscles (those at the thigh, hip, and shoulder) and follow these rules:
- Place your feet comfortably apart, one slightly in front of the other. This ensures a stable, balanced posture.
- Keep your back straight and bend at your knees.
- Grip with your whole hand.
- Keep the weight of the person you are lifting as close to you as possible.
- If you start to lose your balance or grip, lower the casualty, adjust your position or grasp as necessary, and start again.

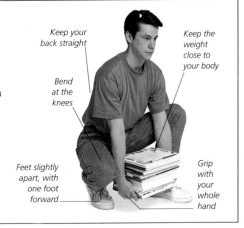

Keep your back straight

Keep the weight close to your body

Bend at the knees

Feet slightly apart, with one foot forward

Grip with your whole hand

CARRIES FOR ONE FIRST AIDER

If no help is available, you can move a casualty using the human crutch method (if they can walk with assistance), or the drag method. Only use the cradle or pick-a-back carries to move lightweight casualties, such as children.

HUMAN CRUTCH

1 Stand on the casualty's injured or weaker side. Pass his arm around your neck, and grasp his hand or wrist with your hand.

2 Pass your other arm around the casualty's waist. Grasp his waistband, or clothing, to support him.

3 Move off on the inside foot. Take small steps, and walk at the casualty's pace. A walking stick or staff may give him additional support. Reassure the casualty throughout.

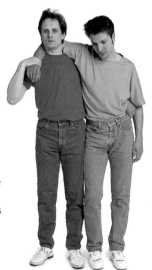

DRAG METHOD

1 Place the casualty's arms across her chest. Crouch behind her, grasp her armpits, and pull.

Keep your back straight

Grasp her wrists firmly

IF the casualty can sit up, cross her arms across her chest, pass your arms under her armpits, grasp her wrists, and pull.

IF she is wearing a jacket, unbutton it and pull it up under her head. Grasp the jacket under the shoulders, and pull.

CRADLE METHOD

1 Squat beside the casualty. Pass one of your arms around the casualty's trunk, above the waist.

Cross her arms across her body

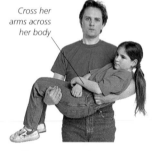

2 Pass your other arm under her thighs. Hug her body towards you, and lift.

PICK-A-BACK

1 Crouch in front of the casualty, with your back to her. Tell her to put her arms around your neck.

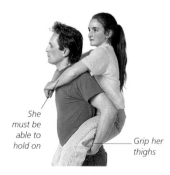

She must be able to hold on

Grip her thighs

2 Grasp the casualty's thighs and rise slowly, keeping your back straight.

CARRIES FOR TWO FIRST AIDERS

Conscious casualties can be moved using the two-handed seat. The fore-and-aft carry can be used to move unconscious casualties, and, in an emergency, may be used to lift a casualty on to a stretcher or carry chair (*see opposite*).

THE TWO-HANDED SEAT

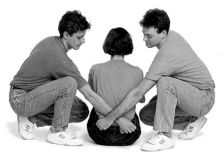

1 Squat facing each other on either side of the casualty. Cross arms behind her back, and grasp her waistband.

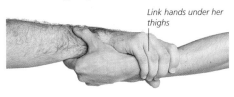

Link hands under her thighs

2 Pass your other hands under the casualty's knees, and grasp each other's wrist. Bring your linked arms up to the middle of the casualty's thighs.

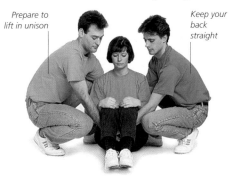

Prepare to lift in unison

Keep your back straight

3 Move in close to the casualty. Keeping your backs straight, rise slowly, and move off together.

THE FORE-AND-AFT CARRY

> DO NOT use this method if the arms or shoulders are injured.

1 Sit the casualty up and put her arms across her chest.

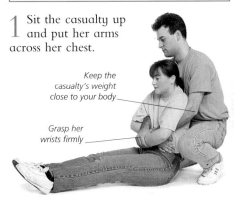

Keep the casualty's weight close to your body

Grasp her wrists firmly

2 Squat behind the casualty. Slide your arms under her armpits and grasp her wrists firmly.

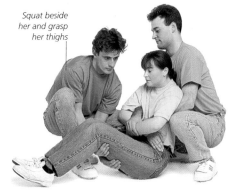

Squat beside her and grasp her thighs

3 Ask your helper to squat beside the casualty and pass his arms under her thighs, taking hold of her legs.

4 Working together, rise slowly, and move off.

CARRY CHAIRS

These are kept in many schools, shops, and workplaces, and are used for moving casualties along passages and up or down stairs. They have wheels, and should have straps for securing the casualty, and are stored folded. You can improvise a carry chair using an ordinary light-weight chair, with broad-fold bandages for straps. Test any chair you use to make sure it will support the casualty's weight.

METHOD

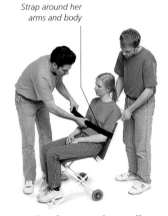

Unfold and test the chair

Footbar

Hand holds

Strap around her arms and body

1 Unfold the chair. Push down on the seat to make sure it can support the casualty's weight.

2 Sit the casualty well back. Cross her arms, put her feet on the bar, and strap her in.

Lifting wheelchairs

In an emergency, casualties in wheelchairs can be transported in their chairs. When going up or down stairs, lift as for a carry chair (*see below*).

Preparing to lift
- Lock the brakes.
- Cross the casualty's arms and secure him or her with straps, or with broad-fold bandages.
- Grasp the chair by secure parts: the handles, or the framework behind the leg-rests. *Do not* grasp the wheels.

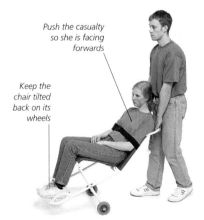

Push the casualty so she is facing forwards

Keep the chair tilted back on its wheels

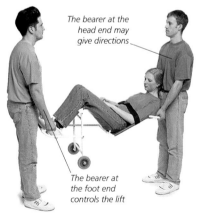

The bearer at the head end may give directions

The bearer at the foot end controls the lift

3 Tilt the chair back on to its wheels, and push forward to move off. When going around corners or over obstacles, pull the chair backwards.

IF you have to go up or down stairs, tilt the chair right back, and ask a helper to lift at the handholds. Always carry the chair with the casualty facing downstairs.

STRETCHERS

These are used to carry casualties to an ambulance or to shelter. The robust standard stretcher may be found at sports grounds, schools, shops, and workplaces. The simpler canvas-and-poles stretcher (*see page 224*) is used to lift a casualty on to a stronger stretcher or ambulance trolley cot. Specialised stretchers include the orthopaedic stretcher (*see page 225*), and the various rescue stretchers (*see page 226*).

General rules for using stretchers

• Inspect stretchers regularly for signs of wear and tear.
• Always test stretchers to make sure they can support a casualty's weight.
• When loading a stretcher, explain to the casualty what is happening.
• Always strap in an unconscious casualty, or one who needs to be transported over any distance.

STANDARD STRETCHERS

The Furley stretcher and the Utila folding stretcher are standard first aid equipment. The Furley stretcher consists of a canvas or plastic sheet, attached to two carrying poles with feet on the underside. Hinged traverses, which may fold in the same direction, or inwards towards each other, keep the stretcher open. The Utila stretcher is similar to the Furley, but is lighter, and more compact when folded.

The Furley stretcher
This collapses widthways, and is stored with the canvas folded over the poles. Some Furley stretchers have straps attached.

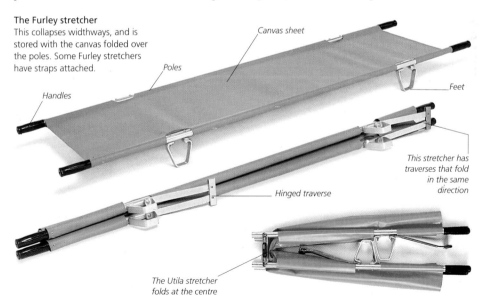

Canvas sheet

Poles

Handles

Feet

This stretcher has traverses that fold in the same direction

Hinged traverse

The Utila stretcher folds at the centre

The Utila stretcher
This more compact version of the Furley stretcher has hinged carrying poles that allow it to fold lengthways. It also has telescopic handles.

OPENING A FURLEY STRETCHER

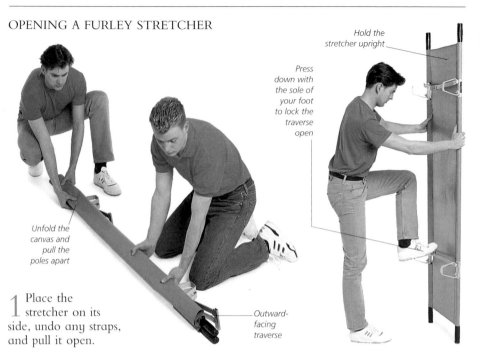

Hold the stretcher upright

Press down with the sole of your foot to lock the traverse open

Unfold the canvas and pull the poles apart

Outward-facing traverse

1 Place the stretcher on its side, undo any straps, and pull it open.

2 Push the outward-facing traverse open with the sole of your foot.

3 Stand the stretcher on its end, and press the other traverse open.

IF both traverses are inward-facing, open both with the stretcher upright.

CLOSING A FURLEY STRETCHER

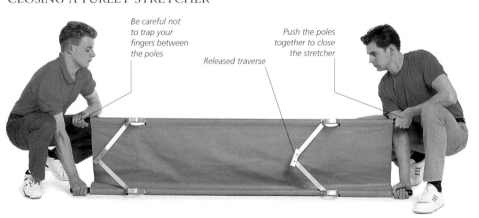

Be careful not to trap your fingers between the poles

Released traverse

Push the poles together to close the stretcher

1 Place the stretcher on its side. Using the sole of your foot, press against the hinge of the traverse until it releases. Do the same for the other traverse.

2 Bring the two poles together, pulling the canvas out from between them. Fold the canvas neatly over the poles. If there are any straps, secure the canvas.

CANVAS-AND-POLES STRETCHER

This is used for lifting a casualty from the ground on to another stretcher, or for transferring a casualty from a stretcher to a trolley cot. It consists of a sheet of canvas or plastic material with handles and side sleeves, and a pair of carrying poles. Spreader bars are inserted between the poles to make the stretcher rigid.

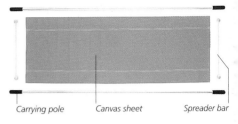

Carrying pole   Canvas sheet   Spreader bar

USING A CANVAS-AND-POLES STRETCHER

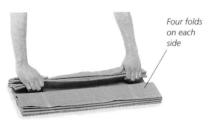

Four folds on each side

1 Concertina-fold one end of the canvas to the middle, making three or four folds. Repeat at the other end.

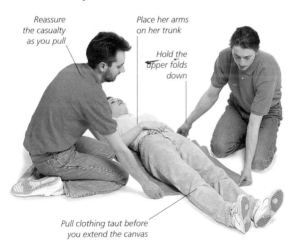

Reassure the casualty as you pull

Place her arms on her trunk

Hold the upper folds down

Pull clothing taut before you extend the canvas

2 Gently slide the folded canvas under the casualty, using the hollow at the small of her back. With one person on either side of the casualty, working together, pull the lower half of the canvas down to her feet.

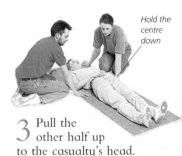

Hold the centre down

3 Pull the other half up to the casualty's head.

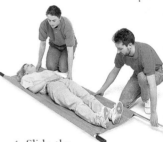

4 Slide the poles up the sleeves of the canvas.

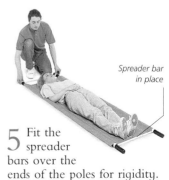

Spreader bar in place

5 Fit the spreader bars over the ends of the poles for rigidity.

ORTHOPAEDIC STRETCHER

Known as the "scoop" stretcher, this is a lightweight device for lifting casualties who must not be moved unduly, or who must be lifted in the position in which they are found (for example, a casualty with spinal injuries). This stretcher splits lengthways into two halves, which are placed on either side of the casualty, then reassembled. Scoop stretchers must not be used to carry a casualty any distance.

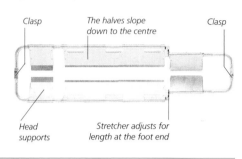

Clasp

The halves slope down to the centre

Clasp

Head supports

Stretcher adjusts for length at the foot end

USING AN ORTHOPAEDIC STRETCHER

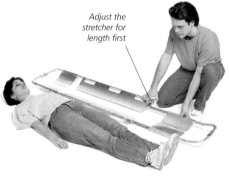

Adjust the stretcher for length first

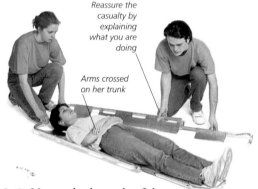

Reassure the casualty by explaining what you are doing

Arms crossed on her trunk

1 Place the stretcher alongside the casualty. Adjust it so that it is slightly longer than the casualty at either end.

2 Uncouple the ends of the stretcher, and ease one half, and then the other, under the casualty.

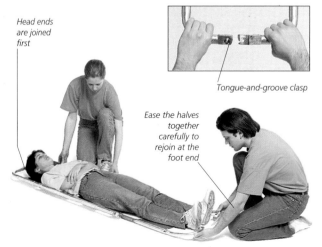

Head ends are joined first

Tongue-and-groove clasp

Ease the halves together carefully to rejoin at the foot end

3 Re-join the stretcher at the head end, while your helper holds the two halves at the foot end firmly in line.

4 Join the foot ends, making sure the casualty's back or buttocks are not pinched.

5 Working together at either end, lift the stretcher very carefully.

6 Place the casualty on a standard stretcher, or trolley cot. Undo the scoop and ease it away.

IMPROVISED STRETCHERS

Although stretchers can be improvised in an emergency, it is always better to wait for specialist help and equipment. If you must move a casualty to shelter, improvise a stretcher using a rigid surface such as a door, hurdle, or advertising hoarding. Alternatively, slide poles through the sleeves of jackets or anoraks (*see right*). Always test the strength of improvised stretchers before you use them.

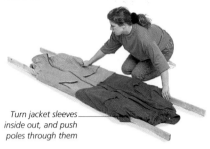

Turn jacket sleeves inside out, and push poles through them

RESCUE STRETCHERS

There are a number of stretchers designed for removing casualties from places that are difficult to get access to, such as cliffs, mines, and tunnels.

The two most commonly used are the Paraguard stretcher and the Neil Robertson (*right*). Both are designed for lifting a casualty vertically or horizontally from awkward places. The casualty is wrapped in the stretcher, and then dragged or lifted to safety. These stretchers should only be used by trained rescue personnel.

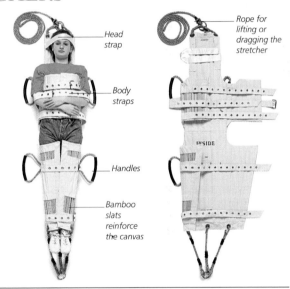

Head strap

Body straps

Handles

Bamboo slats reinforce the canvas

Rope for lifting or dragging the stretcher

INSIDE

TROLLEY COT

Most ambulances carry stretcher trolleys ("trolley cots"). These are fully-adjustable stretcher beds on wheels: the height, tilt, and knee and back rests can be altered to suit the casualty's condition.

Trolley cots have telescopic lifting handles and pull bars, guard rails and straps for safety, and wheels with brakes. They are made of light-weight tubular alloy, but can be heavy when loaded.

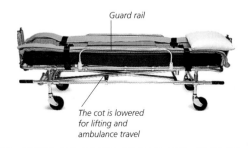

Guard rail

The cot is lowered for lifting and ambulance travel

PREPARING A STRETCHER

Blanketing a stretcher will help keep the casualty warm, and will protect him or her against bumps and jolts. One blanket will do (*see below*), though two is better (*see overleaf*). A canvas carrying sheet may be placed beneath the casualty, so that he or she can be transferred to another stretcher, or to a trolley cot, if necessary.

USING ONE BLANKET

1 Place the open blanket diagonally over the stretcher so that the corners overhang at sides, top, and bottom.

2 Lay the casualty in the centre of the stretcher. Explain to her what you are going to do. Bring the foot overhang over her feet, and tuck it around her ankles.

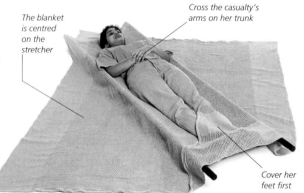

The blanket is centred on the stretcher

Cross the casualty's arms on her trunk

Cover her feet first

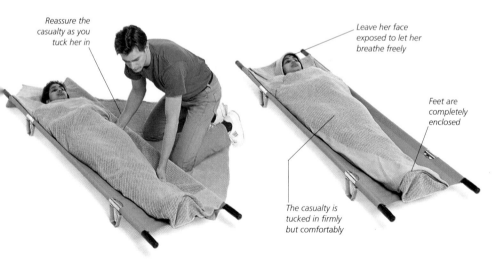

Reassure the casualty as you tuck her in

Leave her face exposed to let her breathe freely

Feet are completely enclosed

The casualty is tucked in firmly but comfortably

3 Bring one side of the blanket over the casualty, and tuck it in securely underneath her.

4 Fold the other side over and tuck it in. Reassure the casualty by explaining what you are doing as you work.

5 Tuck the overhang at the head end round the casualty's head and neck, leaving her face exposed.

IF the casualty is unconscious, or you need to transport her over any distance, make sure she is strapped in securely.

PREPARING A STRETCHER USING TWO BLANKETS

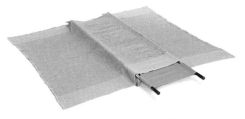

1 Place the first blanket widthways across the stretcher so that one side of the blanket covers the handles at the head end. Centre the blanket on the stretcher.

Making a blanket roll

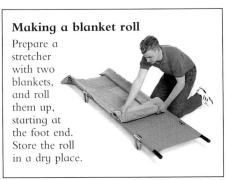

Prepare a stretcher with two blankets, and roll them up, starting at the foot end. Store the roll in a dry place.

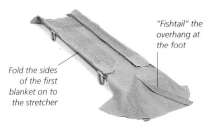

"Fishtail" the overhang at the foot

Fold the sides of the first blanket on to the stretcher

2 Fold the second blanket lengthways into three, and lay it along the stretcher, leaving a two-foot overhang at the foot end. Open out the edges of this overhang diagonally. Concertina-fold the edges of the first blanket on to the sides of the stretcher.

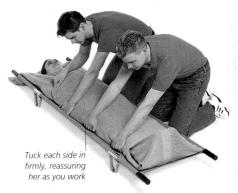

Tuck each side in firmly, reassuring her as you work

4 Bring one side of the blanket over and tuck it in. Repeat with the other side.

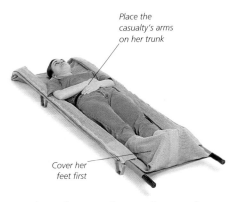

Place the casualty's arms on her trunk

Cover her feet first

3 Place the casualty on the stretcher. Bring the "fishtailed" overhang up over the casualty's feet, and tuck it in around her legs.

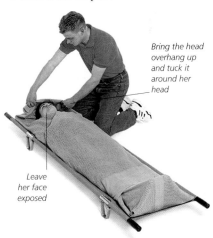

Bring the head overhang up and tuck it around her head

Leave her face exposed

5 Tuck the overhang at the head end around the casualty's head and neck.

LOADING A STRETCHER

The standard way to load a stretcher is to use a canvas-and-poles stretcher (*see page 224*). If you do not have one, you can use the blanket lift illustrated below.

Once the casualty is lifted, she can be lowered on to a stretcher placed either at her feet, or beneath her. If you do not have a blanket, or there are fewer than four bearers, you may use the fore-and-aft carry (*see page 220*). *Do not* lift a casualty who you suspect has a fractured spine; if an immediate risk to life outweighs the danger of movement, use the "log-roll" technique shown on page 156.

BLANKET LIFT

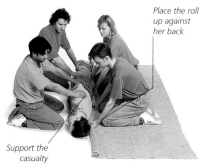

Place the roll up against her back

Support the casualty

1 Roll a blanket lengthways to half its width, and place it alongside the casualty. Roll the casualty on to her side and place the roll against her back.

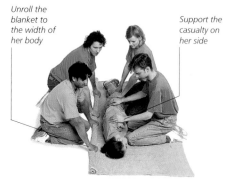

Unroll the blanket to the width of her body

Support the casualty on her side

2 Roll the casualty back over the blanket roll and on to her other side. Unroll enough of the blanket to lay the casualty down flat on it.

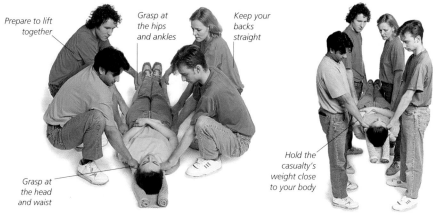

Prepare to lift together

Grasp at the hips and ankles

Keep your backs straight

Grasp at the head and waist

Hold the casualty's weight close to your body

3 Tightly roll the open blanket towards the casualty; the rolls act as handles for the bearers.

4 Two bearers squat on either side of the casualty, at her trunk and legs, and grasp the rolls firmly.

5 On command, all four bearers lift the casualty by leaning back and straightening their knees.

CARRYING A STRETCHER

On the rare occasions when it is necessary to transport a casualty any distance on a stretcher, follow the steps below. The most experienced First Aider co-ordinates the actions of the other bearers, giving commands for each movement.

As a general rule, always carry the casualty feet first. The exceptions are:
• When carrying a casualty with serious limb injuries *down* stairs or an incline.
• When carrying a casualty with hypothermia *down* stairs or an incline.
• Casualties with a stroke or cerebral compression must never be carried with their head lower than their feet.

More advanced techniques for rough ground and obstacles can be found in standard manuals of ambulance aid.

METHOD

1 One bearer stands at each of the four handles.

IF there are only three bearers, two stand at the head, and one at the feet.

2 Each bearer squats and grasps a handle firmly. On command, they all rise together and stand holding the stretcher level.

3 On a further command, the bearers move off on the foot next to the stretcher, taking short steps.

4 To lower the casualty, the bearers stop on command. On a further command, they squat, and lower the stretcher until it rests gently on the ground.

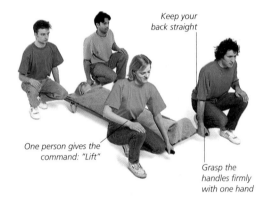

Keep your back straight

One person gives the command: "Lift"

Grasp the handles firmly with one hand

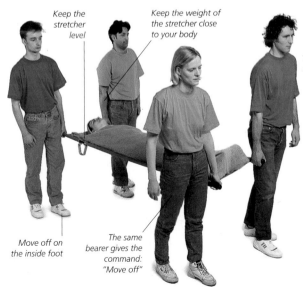

Keep the stretcher level

Keep the weight of the stretcher close to your body

Move off on the inside foot

The same bearer gives the command: "Move off"

Loading ambulances

This is carried out by a trained ambulance crew. Do not assist unless you are asked to do so. You may be asked to support the foot end of the trolley. Be careful not to overlift, as you could throw other bearers off balance.

RESCUE BY HELICOPTER

Rescue helicopters are used for sea and mountain evacuation; smaller helicopter ambulances are increasingly being used in less remote locations. When a helicopter is landing, ground activities are usually co-ordinated by a member of the emergency services, but you should be aware of standard ground-safety precautions (*see below, left*), in case you are asked to help. While the helicopter is landing, protect the casualty from dust and noise; kneel in front of him or her if necessary. If you need to approach the helicopter, follow the safety guidelines listed below.

Standard ground-safety precautions:

• Limit crowd access to a 50-metre perimeter.
• Keep animals under control.
• Ensure that all cigarettes within 50 metres of the landing area are extinguished.
• Remove loose articles, such as broken branches, helmets, or first aid equipment such as stretchers.

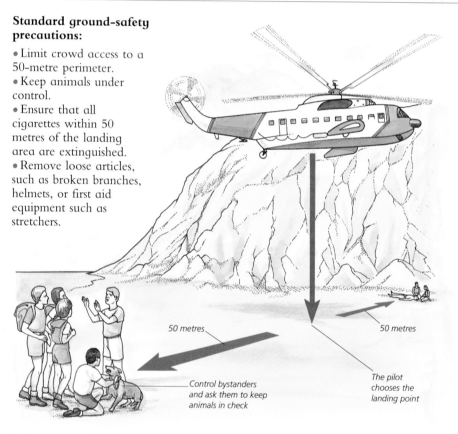

50 metres

50 metres

Control bystanders and ask them to keep animals in check

The pilot chooses the landing point

Safety around helicopters

• Do not move while the helicopter is landing; kneel at the 2 o'clock position to its nose, well back from the rotor blade.
• After the helicopter has landed, wait for a crewman to come to meet you. Do not approach on your own initiative.

• If asked to approach, lower your head and *walk* to the door indicated. Do not approach a helicopter from the rear.
• Do not touch winch lines until they reach the ground; they carry a static electrical charge until earthed.

231

NOTES

INDEX

A

ABC of resuscitation 26
Abdomen:
hernia 184
pains 183
stitch 185
wounds 90
Abdominal thrust 56
Abrasions 76
Absorbed poisons 166
treatment:
household 167
industrial 169
Accidents, road 18-19
Aches:
abdominal pains 183
earache 182
headache 181
toothache 183
Achilles tendon, torn 139
Adhesive dressings 202
Adhesive strapping 202
Afterbirth 196
Aftercare, of casualties 48
Aids, *see* HIV
Airway:
breathing difficulties 62-64
burns to 104
inhalation of fumes 60-61
obstruction 55-59
choking 56-57
opening the 28-29
recovery position 30-31
respiratory system 54
Alcohol:
drunkenness 126
poisoning 170
Allergies 187
anaphylactic shock 71
asthma 63
Alveoli 52
Ambulance dressings 201
Ambulances:
calling for 16
loading 230
trolley cot 226
Amputation 93
Anaemia 67
Anaphylactic shock 71
Angina pectoris 72

B

Animal bites 98
rabies 98
tetanus 96
Ankles:
bandaging 209
fractures 163
sprains 164
Anus, bleeding from 84
Arms:
bandaging 206-207
slings 214-216
bone and muscle injuries:
elbow 149
forearm and wrist 150
hand and fingers 150
upper arm 148
wounds:
amputation 93
bleeding at elbow crease 81
Arteries 66
bleeding from 77
hardening of 67
pulse, the 67
Artificial ventilation:
CPR, in 38
checking for breathing 29
children and babies, for 36-37
face shields, using 32
mouth-to-mouth 32-33
mouth-to-nose 33
mouth-to-stoma 33
Asphyxia 54
Aspirin:
heart attack, and 73
poisoning 168
Assessing casualties:
collapsed casualties 27-29
diagnosis, making a 40-43
top-to-toe survey 44-45
Asthma 63
"Athlete's foot" 188

Babies:
choking 57
convulsions 122
emergency childbirth 189-196
hypothermia 130
resuscitation 36-37
taking pulse 36

Back injuries 153-158
back pain 158
examining for injury 45
spinal injury 154
recovery position in 157
treatment 155-156
Bandages 204-213
applying, general rules of 204
circulation, and 205
reef knots 212
roller bandages 206-209
elbow 208
foot 209
hand 209
knee 208
securing 206
triangular bandages 211-215
foot 212
hand 212
scalp 213
slings, as 214-16
tubular gauze 210
Birth, *see* Childbirth
Bites and stings 97
anaphylactic shock 71
animal bites 98
insect stings 99
marine creatures 100-101
rabies 98
snake bites 102
tetanus 96
Blankets:
blanket lift 229
for stretchers 227-228
storing 228
Bleeding 75-96
treatment:
minor wounds 94
severe wounds 78-79
infection in wounds 96
internal bleeding 83-87
bruises 95
childbirth, following 196
from orifices 84-87
miscarriage 190
shock as a result of 68
types of 77
varicose veins 82
wounds, bleeding from:
abdominal 90
chest 88-89

ACKNOWLEDGMENTS

Contributors to the 6th edition

St. John Ambulance
Mr Andrew K Marsden *Medical Director, Publications*
Mr Jim McKenzie *Training Manager*

St. Andrew's Ambulance Association
Mr Roy Scott *Chief Medical Officer*
Mr George Watt *Director of Training*

British Red Cross
Sir Cameron Moffat *Chief Medical Adviser*
Mr Tony Kemp *Senior Training Officer (First Aid)*

Authors' acknowledgments
The medical authors wish to acknowledge the advice and help of many others, in particular:
Dr Anthony Handley (*Chief Medical Officer, Royal Life Saving Society*); Dr Harry Baker;
Dr David Zideman; Mr Finlay Malcolm; Mr Alan Taylor; Miss Margaret Baker;
Mr Leslie Gibbons; and members of the St. John Ambulance Medical Board.

Managing Editor	Jemima Dunne
Managing Art Editor	Gaye Allen
Project Editor	Louise Abbott
Project Art Editor	Karen Ward
Editor	Victoria Sorzano
Designer	Claire Edwards
Production	Rosalind Priestley
Photography	Steve Gorton
Photographic Assistant	Sarah Ashun
Illustrations	David Ashby, Coral Mula, Gillian Oliver, John Woodcock
Anatomical illustrations	Joanna Cameron

Publishers' acknowledgments
Dorling Kindersley would like to thank: Jim McKenzie for his help with the photo sessions;
Mark Thomson for page make-up; Hilary Bird for the index; Catherine O'Rourke for picture
research; John Newman of St. John Ambulance; St. John Supplies for props; and all members
of Dorling Kindersley staff and friends who posed for the photographs and illustrations.

Photographs: p5 Anthony Crickmay/Camera Press; p100 Oxford Scientific Films/Kathie
Atkinson (*Portuguese man-of-war*), Bruce Coleman Ltd/Dr Frieder Sauer (*weever fish*), Bruce
Coleman Ltd/Neville Fox-Davies (*anemone*); p171 Harry Smith Photo Library.

Typesetting: The Setting Studio/The Alphabet Set
Reproduction: GRB Grafica Fotoreproduztion, Verona, Italy
Printed in England by Jarrold Printing

EMERGENCY
FIRST AID

EMERGENCY ACTION

A-Z OF FIRST AID

EMERGENCY ACTION

In any situation, you must first take three essential steps: *Look for Danger, Remove any Danger, Assess the Casualty.* Only then can you use the chart below to decide on what action you should take.

An unconscious casualty *always* takes priority; even if resuscitation is not necessary, an unconscious person needs immediate attention to ensure that he or she can breathe. Only then should you begin to assess and treat any injuries, and any other, conscious casualties.

Call for help, if necessary, only when it is safe to leave the casualty to do so, *unless* you are alone with a casualty whose heart has stopped (*see below*).

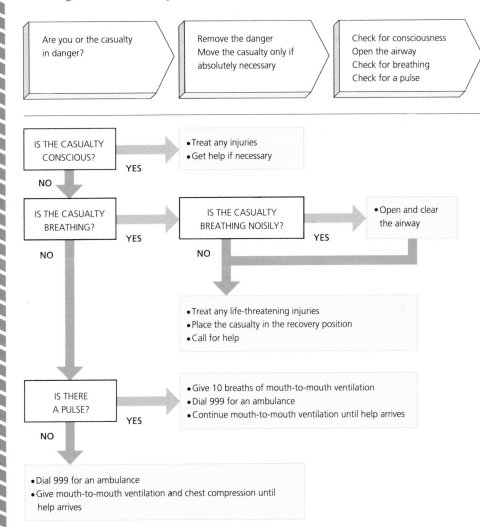

Are you or the casualty in danger?

Remove the danger
Move the casualty only if absolutely necessary

Check for consciousness
Open the airway
Check for breathing
Check for a pulse

IS THE CASUALTY CONSCIOUS?
YES →
• Treat any injuries
• Get help if necessary

NO ↓

IS THE CASUALTY BREATHING?
YES →
IS THE CASUALTY BREATHING NOISILY?
YES →
• Open and clear the airway

NO ↓

NO ↓

• Treat any life-threatening injuries
• Place the casualty in the recovery position
• Call for help

IS THERE A PULSE?
YES →
• Give 10 breaths of mouth-to-mouth ventilation
• Dial 999 for an ambulance
• Continue mouth-to-mouth ventilation until help arrives

NO ↓

• Dial 999 for an ambulance
• Give mouth-to-mouth ventilation and chest compression until help arrives

SEE ALSO: PAGES 28-29 ASSESSING THE CASUALTY

1 *Check for consciousness.*
Shout "Can you hear me?" or "Open your eyes!" Carefully shake the casualty's shoulders. An unconscious casualty will not respond.

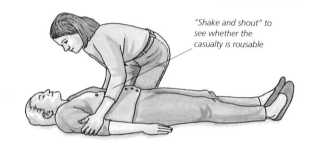

"Shake and shout" to see whether the casualty is rousable

2 *Open an unconscious casualty's air passage.*
Remove any obvious obstruction from the mouth. Place two fingers under the point of the chin, and lift the jaw. At the same time, place your other hand along the casualty's forehead, and tilt her head back.

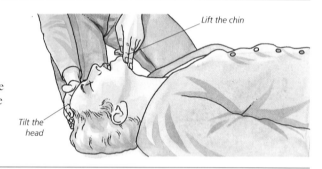

Lift the chin

Tilt the head

3 *Check for breathing.*
Placing your head near the casualty's nose and mouth:
• Look along the chest to see if there is any movement.
• Listen for the sounds of breathing.
• Feel for breath on your cheek.
Check for 5 seconds before deciding breathing is absent.

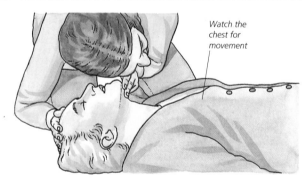

Watch the chest for movement

4 *Check for a pulse.*
With the head tilted back, feel for the Adam's apple with two fingers. Slide your fingers back into the gap between the windpipe and the muscle that runs beside it, and feel for 5 seconds for the carotid pulse.

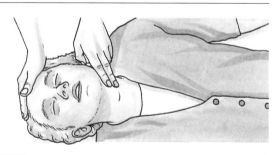

RECOVERY POSITION

SEE ALSO: PAGE 30

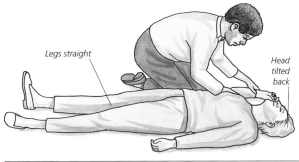

Legs straight

Head tilted back

1 Kneeling beside the casualty, tilt her head and lift her chin to open the airway. Making sure that both her legs are straight, place the arm nearest you out at right–angles to her body, elbow bent, with the palm of the hand uppermost.

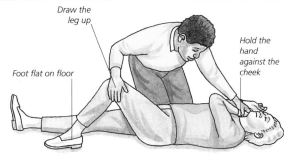

Draw the leg up

Foot flat on floor

Hold the hand against the cheek

2 Bring the far arm across the chest and hold the hand against the casualty's cheek, palm outwards. With your other hand, grasp the farther thigh and pull the knee up, keeping the foot on the ground.

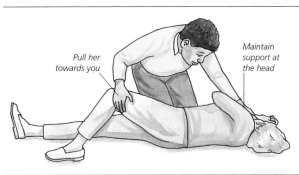

Pull her towards you

Maintain support at the head

3 Keeping the casualty's hand pressed against the cheek with one hand, pull her towards you with the other at the leg.

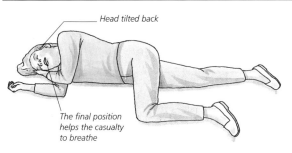

Head tilted back

The final position helps the casualty to breathe

4 Tilt the head back to make sure the airway remains open. Adjust the hand, if necessary, so that the head is well supported. Adjust the uppermost leg so that both the hip and the knee are at right–angles. Check breathing and pulse regularly.

SEE ALSO:
PAGE 32

MOUTH-TO-MOUTH VENTILATION

1 Ensure that the airway is open and the head tilted well back. Pinch the casualty's nostrils closed with your index finger and thumb.

2 Take a deep breath, and seal your lips around the casualty's mouth. Blow into the casualty's mouth until you see the chest rise.

3 Remove your lips and allow the chest to fall. Continue at a rate of 10 breaths per minute.

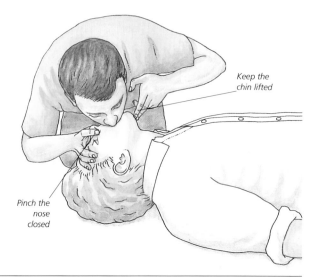

Keep the chin lifted

Pinch the nose closed

SEE ALSO: PAGE 34

CHEST COMPRESSION

1 With the casualty lying flat on a firm surface, place the heel of one hand two finger-widths above the point where his bottom ribs meet his breastbone. Bring the heel of the other hand down over it, and interlock your fingers.

2 With your arms straight, press down vertically on the breastbone, depressing it 4–5cm (1½–2in). Release the pressure. Repeat the compressions at a rate of approximately 80 per minute.

To combine with artificial ventilation: alternate 15 compressions with two breaths until help arrives.

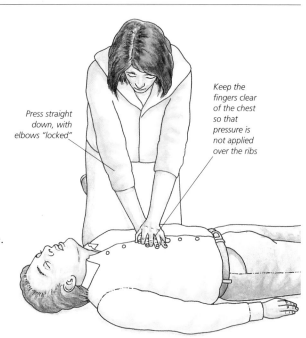

Press straight down, with elbows "locked"

Keep the fingers clear of the chest so that pressure is not applied over the ribs

BLEEDING

SEE ALSO: PAGES 75-96

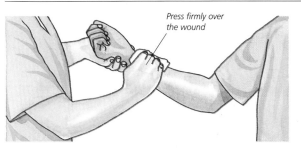

Press firmly over the wound

1 Remove clothing to expose the wound, and press firmly over it with your hand or fingers, preferably over a clean dressing or pad.

DO NOT apply a tourniquet.

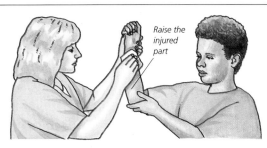

Raise the injured part

2 Maintaining the pressure, raise and support the injured part.

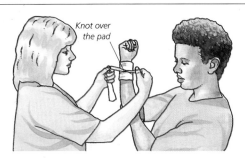

Knot over the pad

3 Bandage the pad firmly in place, but not so tightly that you cut off the blood supply to the limb.

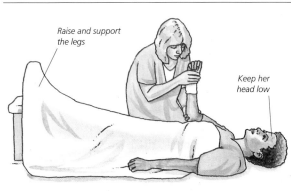

Raise and support the legs

Keep her head low

4 Get appropriate medical help. If bleeding is severe, dial 999 for an ambulance and, keeping the injured part raised and supported, lay the casualty down on a blanket with her legs raised and supported.

If bleeding strikes through the bandage, secure another dressing over the top.

SEE ALSO: PAGES 135–164

BROKEN BONES

1 Tell the casualty to keep still. Steady and support the injured part with your hands.

DO NOT move the casualty unnecessarily.

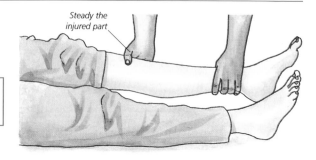

Steady the injured part

2 If there is a wound, control any bleeding by pressing on the wound with a clean dressing or pad. Place soft padding over and around the wound, and bandage the dressing and padding in place.

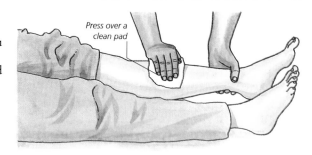

Press over a clean pad

3 For a broken leg, bandage both legs together at knees and ankles, then above and below the injury. For an arm, apply a sling and, if necessary, tie a bandage around the arm and the body, avoiding the injury.

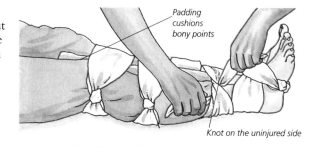

Padding cushions bony points

Knot on the uninjured side

4 Dial 999 for an ambulance. Raise and support the injured part, if possible. Check the circulation in the hand or foot every 10 minutes.

DO NOT give the casualty anything by mouth.

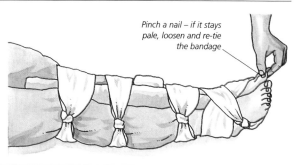

Pinch a nail – if it stays pale, loosen and re-tie the bandage

BURNS

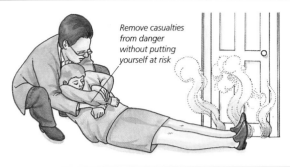

Remove casualties from danger without putting yourself at risk

FIRES

- Immediately dial 999 and ask for the fire brigade.
- Remove casualties from danger if it is safe to do so.
- Do not enter a burning building.
- Do not enter a smoke- or fume-filled room.

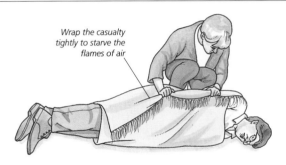

Wrap the casualty tightly to starve the flames of air

CLOTHING ON FIRE

- Do not let the casualty run outdoors.
- Either lay the casualty down, burning side uppermost, and douse him with water, or wrap the casualty tightly in a coat or rug.

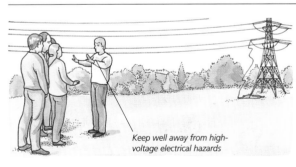

Keep well away from high-voltage electrical hazards

ELECTRICAL INJURIES

Do not approach until:
- You have switched off a domestic current.
- You have been officially informed that a high-voltage current has been switched off and isolated.

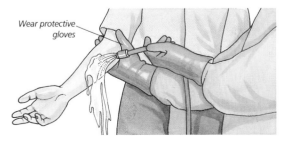

Wear protective gloves

CHEMICAL SPILLS

- Protect yourself from corrosive chemicals.
- Make sure any contaminated rinsing water drains away safely.
- Be aware of the dangers of toxic fumes.

SEE ALSO: PAGES 103-112

BURNS

1 Cool the burn with cold water until the pain is relieved.

> DO NOT delay getting medical help if the burn is severe.

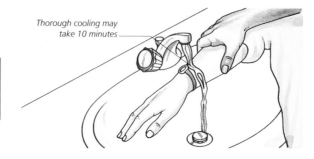

Thorough cooling may take 10 minutes

2 Remove constricting items from the burned area: clothing, belts, shoes, watches, rings, and other jewellery.

> DO NOT remove clothing, or anything else, that sticks to the burn.

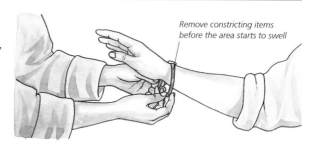

Remove constricting items before the area starts to swell

3 Cover the burn with light, clean, non-fluffy material.

> DO NOT apply cream, ointment, or fat.
>
> DO NOT burst any blisters.

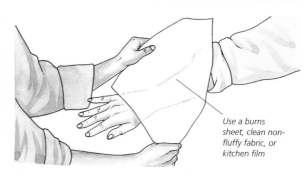

Use a burns sheet, clean non-fluffy fabric, or kitchen film

4 If the burn is large, lay the casualty down and, if possible, raise and support her legs. Check and record breathing and pulse rate every 10 minutes while waiting for medical help or the ambulance to arrive.

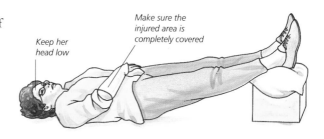

Keep her head low

Make sure the injured area is completely covered

CHOKING

SEE ALSO: PAGE 56

FOR AN ADULT

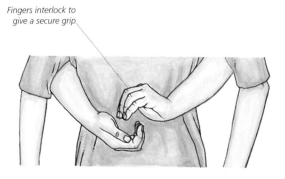

Fingers interlock to give a secure grip

1 Call for an ambulance.

2 Give 6–10 abdominal thrusts: stand behind the casualty and put both arms around her waist, with one hand palm upwards, and the other, palm down.

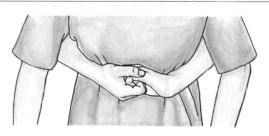

3 Interlock your hands, and pull sharply inwards and upwards below the casualty's ribs. Repeat up to four times.

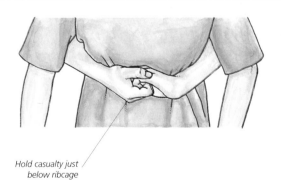

4 If this does not expel the blockage, continue giving abdominal thrusts.

IF the casualty becomes unconscious and is still unable to breathe, follow the treatment on page 56.

Hold casualty just below ribcage

SEE ALSO: PAGE 57

CHOKING

FOR A CHILD

1 Call for an ambulance.

2 Give 6–10 abdominal thrusts: stand behind the casualty and put both arms around his waist, with one hand palm upwards, and the other, palm down.

3 Interlock your hands, and pull sharply inwards and upwards below the casualty's ribs. Repeat 6–10 times.

4 If this does not expel the blockage, keep trying.

IF the casualty becomes unconscious and is still unable to breathe, follow the treatment on page 57.

> DO NOT use your finger to feel blindly down the throat.

FOR A BABY

1 Lay the baby face down along your forearm and give five sharp slaps on the back. If this fails, turn her face up on your arm, or on your lap; give five sharp thrusts to the lower breast-bone, using two fingers only.

2 Check the mouth and remove any object you can see. Repeat the whole process as often as necessary.

3 If the baby becomes unconscious, begin resuscitation and call an ambulance.

> DO NOT use the abdominal thrust technique on a baby.

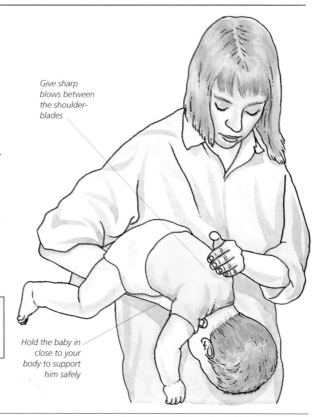

Give sharp blows between the shoulder-blades

Hold the baby in close to your body to support him safely

EYE INJURY

SEE ALSO: PAGE 91
PAGES 111-112

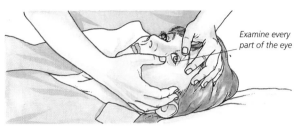

Examine every part of the eye

1 Lay the casualty on her back, and support her head so that it is as still as possible. Examine the affected eye.

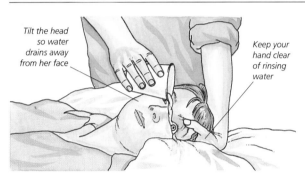

Tilt the head so water drains away from her face

Keep your hand clear of rinsing water

2 Irrigate the eye, if appropriate, to remove a harmful chemical or floating grit.

> DO NOT irrigate an eye with a wound, or a foreign body lodged in or sticking to the eyeball.

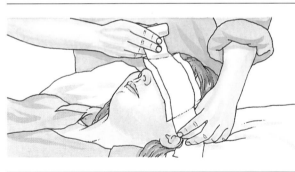

3 Cover the eye, preferably with a sterile eye pad. Bandage the pad firmly in place, covering both eyes to prevent eye movement. Reassure the casualty before you blindfold her.

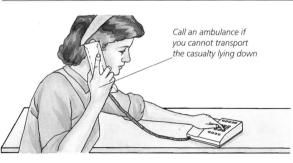

Call an ambulance if you cannot transport the casualty lying down

4 Take or send the casualty to hospital.

SEE ALSO: UNCONSCIOUSNESS, PAGE 256
PAGES 117–119

HEAD INJURY

1 If there is a scalp wound, replace any skin flaps and, using a clean pad, press down firmly and evenly over the wound.

> DO NOT touch the wound with your fingers.

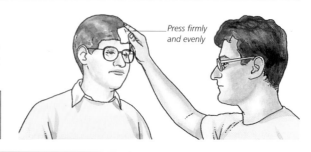

Press firmly and evenly

2 Once bleeding is controlled, hold the pad in place with a bandage.

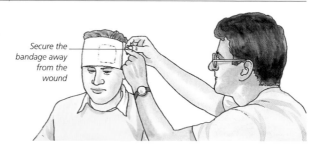

Secure the bandage away from the wound

3 Check the casualty's level of response by asking simple, direct questions. If consciousness is impaired for more than 3 minutes, dial 999 for an ambulance. Record breathing and pulse rate, and level of response, every 10 minutes.

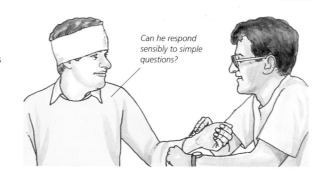

Can he respond sensibly to simple questions?

4 Lay the casualty down, with his head and shoulders raised and supported. Take or send him to hospital in this position.
  If he becomes unconscious, place him in the recovery position (*page 244*) and dial 999 for an ambulance.

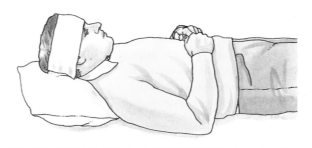

HEART ATTACK

SEE ALSO: PAGE 73

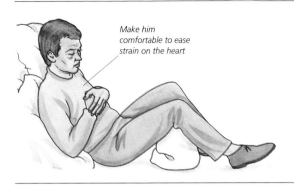

Make him comfortable to ease strain on the heart

1 Make the casualty comfortable. A half-sitting position, with his knees bent and supported, is often the best.

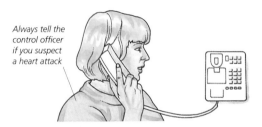

Always tell the control officer if you suspect a heart attack

2 Dial 999 for an ambulance, and tell the control officer that you suspect a heart attack. If the casualty asks for his doctor, call the doctor too.

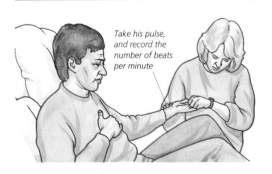

Take his pulse, and record the number of beats per minute

3 Reassure the casualty, and keep a constant check on breathing and pulse, until help arrives. Be ready to resuscitate if necessary.

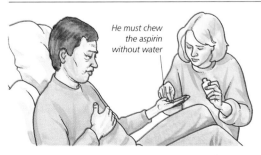

He must chew the aspirin without water

4 If you have ordinary aspirin available and the casualty is conscious, give him one tablet and tell him to chew it slowly.

SEE ALSO: PAGES 165-172 # SWALLOWED POISONS

1 Check that there is no vomit or foreign matter in the casualty's mouth, and that he can breathe.

DO NOT try to make the casualty vomit.

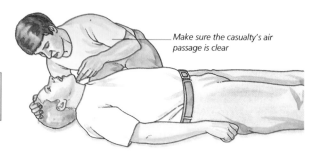

Make sure the casualty's air passage is clear

2 Look for signs of chemical burning in or around the casualty's mouth. If there is burning, give him cold water or milk to sip.

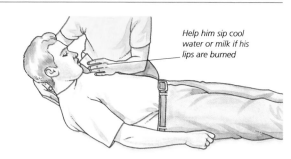

Help him sip cool water or milk if his lips are burned

3 Call a doctor, or dial 999 for an ambulance. Try to identify what the casualty has swallowed, and tell the doctor or ambulance control officer.

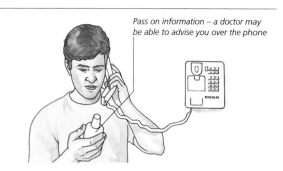

Pass on information – a doctor may be able to advise you over the phone

4 If the casualty becomes unconscious, place him in the recovery position (*page 244*).

Head tilted back, supported by the hand

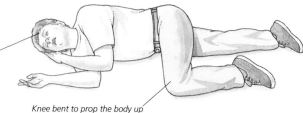

Knee bent to prop the body up

UNCONSCIOUSNESS

SEE ALSO: PAGES 114-126

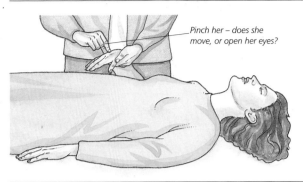

Pinch her – does she move, or open her eyes?

1 Lift the casualty's chin and tilt her head to open the air passage. Check that breathing and pulse are present. Assess her level of response by speaking loudly close to her ear, and pinching the back of her hand. Write down your findings.

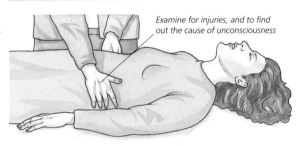

Examine for injuries, and to find out the cause of unconsciousness

2 Examine her quickly and thoroughly, and treat any serious injuries. Try to establish the cause of unconsciousness.

DO NOT move the casualty unnecessarily.

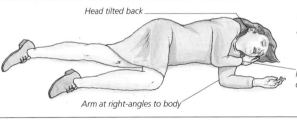

Head tilted back

Hand under cheek

Arm at right-angles to body

3 Place the casualty in the recovery position.

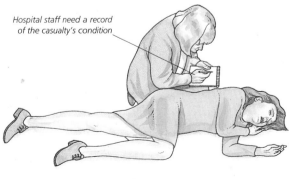

Hospital staff need a record of the casualty's condition

4 If the casualty does not regain conscious-ness in three minutes, dial 999 for an ambulance. Record the casualty's breathing and pulse rate, and level of response, every 10 minutes. Stay with the casualty until the ambulance arrives. Pass on your notes.